Health and Sickness: the Choice of Treatment

Health and Sickness
The Choice of Treatment

*Perception of Illness and Use of Services in
an Urban Community*

M. E. J. WADSWORTH, W. J. H. BUTTERFIELD
and R. BLANEY

*Department of Medicine, Guy's Hospital
Medical School*

TAVISTOCK PUBLICATIONS

First published in 1971
By Tavistock Publications Limited
11 New Fetter Lane, London EC4
Printed in Great Britain
In 10 point 2 point leaded Times New Roman
By The Camelot Press Ltd, London and Southampton

SBN 422 73360 1

Distributed in the USA
by Barnes & Noble, Inc.

For Jane, Isabel, and Brenda

Contents

Contents

Acknowledgements

This study was undertaken initially with a continuing grant from the King Edward's Hospital Fund for London. Later, support was kindly provided by the Board of Governors of Guy's Hospital, and almost all of the computer time was made freely available by the Biophysics Research Unit of the Medical Research Council. Most of the computer programmes were written by Miss Jane Arnott (later Mrs M. E. J. Wadsworth) and she was helped by the earlier work of Mr J. H. Fuller and Mr I. C. F. Oak of Elliott Medical Automation. More recently, programming help and advice were provided by Miss Margaret Elliott and Miss Susannah Brown gave statistical advice.

For the collection and accuracy of the data about complaints and how people managed them we are much indebted to the interviewers and coders, Miss Elizabeth Day, Miss Mary Scott-Brown, Miss Rosemary Ashley, Miss Sheila McKelvey, Mr A. Hasler, Mr C. Hall, Mr J. Monroe, Mr M. Edwards, and Mr P. St John, all of whom spent many cold evenings patiently cycling around the boroughs and carrying out interviews, often rather long ones, in houses and flats.

We are much indebted to Mrs Kay Hasler for her original work with and interpretation of our attempts at drawing figures and diagrams. *Figure 1* on p. 6 is reproduced from *Uses of Epidemiology* by J. N. Morris, by kind permission of the publishers, E. & S. Livingstone. Special thanks are also due to the many secretaries who have worked patiently on the manuscript at various stages of its preparation, and to the publishers for their patience.

Finally, but by no means least, we are very grateful indeed to colleagues at Guy's Hospital in London, in the Department of General Practice in Edinburgh, in the Medical Research Council in London, and in the University of Leeds (where M.E.J.W. presented some of these data as part of the requirements for the degree of Master of Philosophy), all of whom have given much sound advice, help, and useful criticism during the course of the work.

Foreword

In 1962 a study group was set up in the Department of Medicine at Guy's Hospital Medical School to carry out a study of a sample of the population living in the immediate neighbourhood of the hospital, that is in the old London County Council boroughs of Bermondsey and Southwark.

The group's work began with an investigation of the use of outpatient services by the general practitioners in Bermondsey and Southwark.[1] The second phase consisted of a study of new outpatients referred to Guy's Hospital over a period of four months in 1963.[2, 3, 4, 5, 6] At the same time data were collected for a comparative study of outpatient services in a London hospital group, and a group of provincial hospitals, and this was reported by the Nuffield Provincial Hospitals Trust.[7]

This present report covers the third part of the study, which aimed to examine another aspect of the relationship between the medical services and the boroughs of Bermondsey and Southwark.* It is concerned not just with complaints or conditions that are already receiving medical care, but with the management, both medical and otherwise, of all complaints experienced by a random sample of the population of the two boroughs. This was undertaken because of our belief that information forms a vital background – in the present circumstances of changes in the prevailing pattern of illness and changes in the population structure and way of life – to the understanding of 'demand' for services providing medical care.

* A summary of all three studies and a report on a pilot study of this third part is given in (8).

REFERENCES

1. ACHESON, R. M., BARKER, D. J. P., & BUTTERFIELD, W. J. H. (1962). How General Practitioners use Outpatient Services in two London Boroughs. *Brit. med. J.* **2** 1315.
2. BLANEY, R. (1965) Factors Determining Attendance at the O.P.D. of a London Teaching Hospital. Unpublished M.D. thesis, Queen's University of Belfast.
3. ACHESON, R. M., BLANEY, R., BUTTERFIELD, W. J. H., CHAMBERLAIN, JOCELYN, & SCOTT-BROWN, MARY. (1963) Factors influencing Referrals to the Outpatients Department of a London Teaching Hospital. *Brit. J. prev. soc. Med.* **17** 81–84.
4. CHAMBERLAIN, JOCELYN, ACHESON, R. M., BUTTERFIELD, W. J. H., & BLANEY, R. (1966) The Population Served by the Outpatient Department of a London Teaching Hospital: A Study of Guy's. *Med. Care* **4** 81–88.
5. BLANEY, R., ACHESON, R. M., BUTTERFIELD, W. J. H., & CHAMBERLAIN, JOCELYN (1966) Outpatient Services of the London Teaching Hospitals 1951–1961: An Analysis of Official Statistics. *Med. Care* **4** 89–93.
6. BUTTERFIELD, W. J. H., WADSWORTH, M. E. J., & BLANEY, R. (1966) A London Teaching Hospital, in *Problems and Progress in Medical Care*, II 123–152. Oxford University Press for the Nuffield Provincial Hospitals Trust.
7. CHAMBERLAIN, JOCELYN (1966) Two Non-Teaching Hospitals in South East England, in *Problem and Progress in Medical Care*, II 43–76. Oxford University Press for The Nuffield Provincial Hospitals Trust.
8. BUTTERFIELD, W. J. H. (1965) The Orientation of the Consultant towards the New Approach to Public Health. *Public Health* **79** 218–226.

CHAPTER I

Introduction

For many years there have been basically two very different attitudes to medical practice as a national welfare service with free choice of a doctor and free access to consult him at will. The benefits and disadvantages of both the state and the privately based systems have scarcely been clarified in 'hard' terms and have usually been expressed as hopes or fears. These two sorts of attitude may be summarized in words taken from famous practical social philosophers and commentators.

The first attitude is a fear that state-subsidized medicine and free choice of and access to a doctor for everybody would result in unutterable chaos, with the medical services swamped with trivial complaints, or as it was once called 'Pharmacomania'. The Webbs commented that:

'Any such system [i.e. publicly subsidized system with free choice of doctor] would lead, not only to a most serious inroad upon the work and emoluments of the private practitioner, but also to an extravagent expenditure of public funds on popular remedies and 'medical extras', without obtaining in return for this enlarged 'Medical Relief', greater regularity of life or more hygienic habits in the patient' [1910].[1]

Fears of the 'abuse' of the free hospital outpatient departments (i.e. their use by patients who either could afford to pay for treatment or were hypochondriacs or malingerers) – and these departments were the forerunners of the present general practitioner service – were common even in 1869.[2, 3] Today, the dangers of 'frivolous demands from a small number of people'[4] are commonly mentioned as a hindrance to the proper functioning of general medical practice, and indeed were so even before the introduction of the National Health Service.

'The present status of the general practitioner is unsatisfactory because he is too overburdened with routine work to exercise judgement and to act as an effective health adviser' [1937].[5]

The second attitude is very different. This consists of the hope, expressed especially often at the time of proposal and inauguration of the National Health Service, that free access to medical care for all should act as a system for the early identification, and thus reduction, of disease in the community. For example, in 1943 *The Times* predicted in an editorial that

'any health budget will show on the credit side a substantial saving to the nation by the reduction of disease.'[6]

Similarly, in the famous *White Paper* of 1942, Beveridge wrote that

'there will be actually some development of the service, and as a consequence of this development a reduction in the number of cases requiring it.'[7]

Both these views try to predict something about the *demand* for medical care or the level of expectation of medical care under a national health service. Obviously, it would be invaluable to be able to say that one or other of them was correct. However, since they were expressed, a number of intervening factors have considerably complicated the situation. Nevertheless, both of these attitudes are still commonly expressed. In order to discuss, at the present time, the problems of predicting the demand for health services a review of these factors is necessary.

The two chief factors are the changing pattern of disease and the trends in the population structure of the British Isles.

First, the demographic factor. Using March's interpretation of the intercensal changes from 1871 to 1961, it is possible to summarize the most relevant movement, namely the changes in age distribution, in age at marriage and retirement, in family size, and in patterns of employment. The rise in the proportion of elderly persons in the community is well known, although it is necessary to remember that 'any discussion of old-age is immediately made difficult by the problem of adequately defining the term "old".[8] Less well known, as Marsh indicates, is the 'fundamental change' in the balance between the young and the middle-aged. 'By 1961 . . . the 0–19 group is now much larger than the 20–39 group, but unlike the nineteenth century the 20–39 age group is still not as large as the 40–59 age group.'[9] Where marriage is concerned, a larger proportion of persons are married than ever before, marriage tends to take place earlier, and family size is smaller than in the late nineteenth and early twentieth centuries.[10] The proportion of retired workers has risen, and the proportion of clerical and other sedentary workers has also increased.[11, 12]

These factors, along with changes in dietary habits,[13] with increased cigarette-smoking, and with increasing mechanization discouraging physical exercise at both work and leisure, are, with other features of life-styles and environmental influences, commonly postulated as having affected the changing pattern of disease. More sensitive diagnostic methods, and advances in pharmacy, in vaccination and immunization, and in many other technical and medical-scientific fields have been similarly influential.

As a result, the decline in infectious diseases has not been accompanied, as many people had hoped, by a great reduction in the numbers of sick persons in the community, but by a change in the types of common disorder. As 'the old emergencies, lobar pneumonia, emphysema, mastoiditis, have disappeared', so 'the stresses of affluence, obesity, varicose veins, haemorrhoids',[14] etc., have become increasingly important. Morris has called this process the *onion principle*:

'The death rate falls, and questions of morbidity assume a new importance. With the decline of the crowd diseases, other infections and non-infectious diseases predominate. Lessen physical deprivation, and widespread emotional impoverishment and social incompetence are exposed. Reduce physical disease, and problems of mental health can no longer be ignored. When environmental casualties are controlled, genetic failures receive more attention.'[15]

In addition Logan,[16] Butterfield,[17] and Morris assert that not only is the pattern of disease changing but also expectation of or demand for medical care is rising.

'The supply of health services sharpens perception of need and raises expectations, i.e. produces more cases; social security benefits as said raise the rate of declared incapacity. Disability from

3

byssinosis has increased fifty-fold because of changes in the compensation law.'[18]

Thus far, at any rate, it would seem that both the attitudes set out at the beginning of this chapter are in some degree justified. As some feared, there has been an increase in the usage of medical care services. Guillebaud (1956)* and Willinck (1959),† for example, both bear witness to this. At the same time, as others hoped, the incidence of some diseases – e.g. tuberculosis – has been very much reduced.

Now there are, however, two further complicating factors that obscure and change this fairly clear picture.

First, screening, or the early detection of disease. Diagnostic methods for the discovery of illness at the presymptomatic or biochemical stage are being developed and improved. Studies using such methods have shown that in some conditions there exists a much greater reservoir of unrecognized ill health than of disease brought to medical attention. Thus, for example, in an average British general practice of 2,250 persons, it has been estimated that for every 8 persons presenting in one year with diabetes a further 69 will have 'latent diabetes', which is not brought to the doctor but may be detected on survey; for the 89 patients presenting with psychiatric disorder, a further 71 will have 'conspicuous psychiatric morbidity'; and for the 5 presenting with ischaemic heart disease, a further 15 may be detected on survey.[19] The results of these sorts of survey have led to the formulation of the *iceberg concept*, which describes unrecognized and untreated disease in the community as the submerged part of the iceberg, and the recognized and treated illness as the small 'tip'.

The iceberg concept and the development of screening techniques have two important implications. In view of the existence of the iceberg and of screening methods it is not unreasonable to postulate the imminence of effective methods of treating disease that has been detected very early in its course. This would indeed be the sort of contribution to the advancement of preventive medicine which Beveridge anticipated. But, in order to achieve it, undoubtedly some-

---

* Chairman of the committee set up to examine the rise in expenditure on pharmaceuticals.

† Chairman of the committee set up to examine future medical manpower needs.

4

thing of the order of a new branch of the National Health Service would be necessary, which would also require a new army of supportive paramedical staff.

And not only would a new branch of the National Health Service be necessary, but the whole concept of the doctor/patient relationship would need to be reviewed, for early detection means that the doctor must initiate the episode of consultation, a task at present almost always the responsibility of the patient. McKeown has summarized this as follows:

> 'When the patient seeks medical advice the doctor's position ethically, is relatively simple: he undertakes to do his best with the knowledge and resources available to him . . . The position is quite different in screening, when a doctor or public medical authority takes the initiative in investigating the possibility of illness or disability in persons who have not complained of signs or symptoms. There is then a presumptive undertaking, not merely that abnormality will be identified if it is present, but that those affected will derive benefit from subsequent treatment or care. This commitment is at least implicit . . .'[20]

At present very little is known about the reception such a service would receive. One study[21] has shown that two-thirds of persons might be interested to use such facilities, but how much this reaction might change with an increase in availability of tests is open to speculation. This, briefly, is the first complicating factor in the original picture of demographic change and of movements in the prevailing pattern of disease.

The second factor concerns the individual patient, and is not of such recent origin as screening and the iceberg concept. It is the concept of disease causation. In his discussion of this, with particular reference to ischaemic heart disease, Morris says:

> '. . . its manifold associations, variety of presentation and unpredictable outcome have accustomed the physician to think of ischaemic heart disease in "multi-factorial" terms, of an extending complex of events in, and interactions between, persons and their environments.
>
> Many pathologies then are involved in ischaemic heart disease; it is the product of many causes, and we have to think of the

patterns these form. . . . it is even conceivable that there is no specific agent of ischaemic heart disease.'[22]

Similarly, in discussing cigarette-smoking:

'Cigarette smoking seems now to be a leading cause of chronic bronchitis, but last century there was a lot of the disease – and no cigarettes. The driven, striving, competitive person surely was familiar in Victorian England, but it is quite conceivable that he rarely suffered from ischaemic heart disease. Such refutation would not dispose of these hypotheses. Other *patterns* of causes presumably were operating last century, the epidemic constitution was different, other things never are equal.'[23]

In his conclusion Morris notes that 'a main lesson of ecology and of social science is about interrelatedness – one effect cannot be produced without a lot of others, intended and unintended'.[24] An indication of the importance of this so-called *multiple-causation theory* is instanced in the establishment in Tecumseh, Michigan, of an investigation 'to study a complete natural community including the population and its biological, physical, and social environment'.[25] It is again Professor Morris who summarizes most concisely with the diagram shown at *Figure 1*.[26] Whereas (1) and (2) have been traditionally regarded as coordinates of overriding importance in seeking

Figure 1   The major elements in the multiple causation of disease

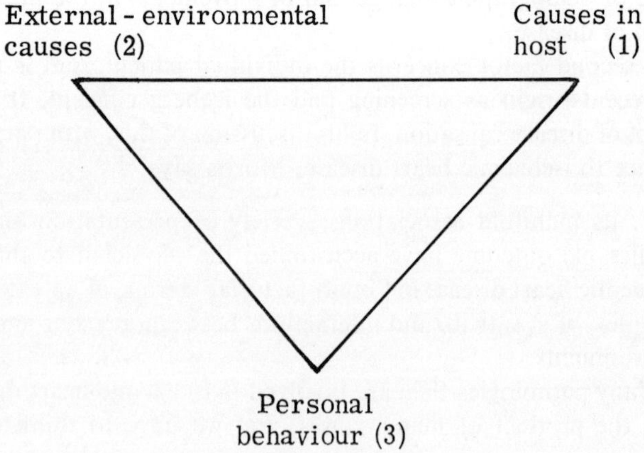

External - environmental
causes (2)

Causes in
host   (1)

Personal
behaviour (3)

6

for causes of disease, the changing pattern of disease has (among many other things) helped to introduce the importance of (3), and thus consideration of the total *life-style*.

From all of the foregoing two important points emerge. First, that the original conflicting and popularly expressed views with which this chapter began are such gross oversimplifications of the situation that there can be no question of complete 'correctness' or otherwise of either of them. It is neither simply a case of the general national state of health improving, and therefore reducing the numbers of patients, nor is it just that patients are presenting with more trivial complaints more frequently. Disease patterns are changing, and the emphasis, in disease presented to medical care, is away from the acute, episodic type of illness, and towards the chronic conditions requiring long-term management and surveillance.

Second, it emerges that both for clear understanding of disease processes and for the assistance of planners in the situation of structural changes in the health services, further study of the present nebulous area of the effects of individual life-styles, and of individuals initial management and interpretation of complaints, is necessary.

The present investigation, therefore, set out to ascertain the extent of disease (i.e. deviation, as defined by each respondent, from his normal state of health) in a study population, and to describe the measures taken to alleviate or cure these complaints so that the proportion referred to medical care might be estimated. This procedure was felt to cover some of the preliminaries for better understanding of the role of the individual in determining the picture of the general national state of health, and of the level of demand for medical care, the necessity for which this introduction endeavours to describe.

REFERENCES

1. WEBB, S., & WEBB, B. (1910) *The State and the Doctor*, p. 230. Longmans Green, London.
2. *Lancet* (1869) Investigation into the Administration of the Out-Patient Department of the London Hospitals, p. 435.
3. WADSWORTH, M. E. J. (1968) Towards Perspective in Medical Care Research. *Soc. Econ. Admin.* **2** 106.
4. MEDICAL SERVICES REVIEW COMMITTEE (1962) *A Review of the Medical Services in Britain* Para. 207, 57.

5. POLITICAL AND ECONOMIC PLANNING (1937) *Report on the British Health Services*, p. 25.
6. *The Times* (1943) From a leading article on proposals for a comprehensive medical service. 7 August, p. 5.
7. *Social Insurance and Allied Services* (The Beveridge Report) (1942). para 270 Cmnd. 6404, HMSO, London.
8. MARSH, D. C. (1967) *The Changing Social Structure of England & Wales 1871–1961*, p. 23. Routledge & Kegan Paul, London.
9. Op. cit. MARSH D. C. (1967) 26.
10. Op. cit. MARSH D. C. (1967) 32–39.
11. Op. cit. MARSH D. C. (1967) 133.
12. Op. cit. MARSH D. C. (1967) 158–160.
13. YUDKIN, J. (1967) Evolutionary and dietary changes in carbohydrates. *Amer. J. clin. Nutn.* **20**. 108.
   SUKHATME, P. V. (1967) Personal communication to W. J. H. Butterfield published in *Priorities in Medicine* (1968) Nuffield Provincial Hospitals Trust, London.
14. BUTTERFIELD, W. J. H. (1964) Foreword in *New Frontiers in Health*, p. 3. Office of Health Economics, London.
15. MORRIS, J. N. (1967) *Uses of Epidemiology*, p. 14. Livingstone, Edinburgh.
16. LOGAN, R. F. L. (1965) *Trends in the Study of Morbidity and Mortality*. WHO, Geneva.
17. BUTTERFIELD, W. J. H. (1968) *Priorities in Medicine*, p. 22. Nuffield, London.
18. Op. cit. MORRIS, J. N. (1967) 15.
19. Op. cit. MORRIS, J. N. (1967) 122.
20. MCKEOWN, T. (1968) Validation of Screening Procedures, in *Screening in Medical Care*, 2. Nuffield Provincial Hospitals Trust, Oxford University Press, London.
21. CARTWRIGHT, A. (1967) *Patients and their Doctors*. Routledge and Kegan Paul, London.
22. Op. cit. MORRIS, J. N. (1967) 173.
23. Op. cit. MORRIS, J. N. (1967) Note on p. 260.
24. Op. cit. MORRIS, J. N. (1967) 268.
25. FRANCIS, T., & EPSTEIN, F. N. (1965) Tecumseh, Michigan, p. 333. *Milbank Memorial Fund Quarterly*.
26. Op. cit. MORRIS, J. N. (1967) 192.

CHAPTER 2

The Problem, and a Brief Review of the Literature

'*Morbidity* is but one illustration of the modern community's need to know itself, a need whose wide recognition—anew—represents a striking change in the contemporary climate of opinion. A tragic and shameful growth of homeless families in London was suddenly exposed late in 1961. The country entered the recent war with 9 per cent of the population over 65 years of age, and no problem; at its close there were 10 per cent, and Old Age was suddenly The Social Problem of The Century – but recognized too late to affect the 1948 legislation. From the condition of the recruits in the Boer War to the thalidomide calamity . . . , and not forgetting the boy whose death led to the Children Act, society is liable to be caught by surprise, and not in all instances inevitably, . . . The more complex a society, the more does it need an inquisitive intelligence service to diagnose itself . . . and to probe the consequences of trends and policies.'[1]

Exactly why *morbidity* has recently become of great importance may be illustrated by reference to the brief discussion in Chapter 1 of the changing pattern of disease, and more specifically with the assistance of *Figure 2*. This diagram illustrates the disease process, with a continuous movement of individuals from a state of perfect health (upper part of figure) to one of manifest ill health (lower part). The changing pattern of disease (together with many other things) has affected the dimension of each of the component parts of the figure. As the incidence of acute illness and of infections is reduced by public health measures and by the use of antibiotics, so chronic disease becomes more widespread, and the common illnesses no longer have easily recognizable onsets. The predominance of acute illness has given way to a common pattern of illnesses characterized by their episodic nature and often, too, by their insidious onset. Anxiety, obesity, bronchitis, diabetes, and varicose veins have been cited as examples of such conditions.[2]

Figure 2   Model of the disease process

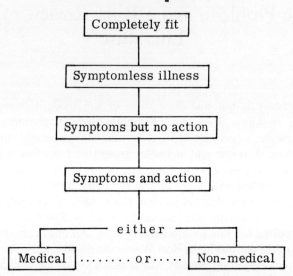

This change shows itself in the working of health services by the tendency for hospital departments, both inpatient and outpatient, and for general practitioners to see more patients many times for short periods, rather than smaller numbers of patients on fewer occasions for longer periods. The change is undoubtedly also associated with complaints from doctors of patients wasting their time with trivia – as one doctor recently wrote in a national newspaper, 'we have already quite enough of shamming illness'.[3]

For some individuals, these features – an episodic pattern and an insidious onset – may well help to bring about certain types of behaviour. Both features may lead some persons to try self-medication, which would certainly not be an unreasonable course of management for the sort of minor symptoms often associated with the beginning of a chronic illness. In addition, an episodic pattern may offer a degree of reassurance, when intervals of normal health occur between episodes of complaints.

In order to describe the real distribution of the divisions set out in

10

the hypothetical diagram (*Figure 2*), the present study set out to discover, in a randomly selected population, all complaints suffered and every measure taken, both medically and non-medically pre-scribed, to manage them.

Clearly, the basis for such an investigation is an assessment of total morbidity in the study population. Available clinical statistics, however, usually begin only at the point of medical diagnosis, and give no information on what preceded this event. Thus a special data-collection had to be carried out in order to fulfil the objective of obtaining a complete picture of all complaints, and of all measures taken for them, that had occurred in the study population over a specified period of time. A clinical examination and assessment of each respondent was not felt to be necessary,* since interest was focused not on the diagnosis but on the person's own management and interpretation of complaints. Considerable care in the interpreta-tion of results is therefore necessary. As Logan and Brooke have pointed out,[4] reporting of complaints in response to a questionnaire does not necessarily indicate extant illness, and in the present work it certainly does not indicate the severity of any complaint. Similarly, it does not necessarily show a medically correct morbidity picture, for many complaints may well be incorrectly categorized. For example, a complaint presented at interview as backache may be due to renal disorder or gynaecological disease or may be of ortho-paedic origin. A comment on this appears in Chapter 4.

Despite these two qualifying points, the method employed is not without benefits. Respondents' reporting specifically about their health complaints uniquely shows how much ill health† is felt and how many complaints suffered, and thus permits assessment of the extent of unreported illness, both lay-treated and not treated. This means that data collected may be fairly interpreted as reflecting individuals' own decisions as to how to manage their complaints.

There is a considerable literature both in the social sciences and in medicine to provide guideposts and precedents for this kind of

---

* Although, clearly, it would have added, at considerable expense, an interesting additional dimension, and there has subsequently been a medical examination of 2,000 persons in the borough by the local Medical Officer of Health, which is discussed in Chapter 10.

† Following the definition used by Hinkle *et al.*[5] a complaint of ill health is 'any departure from an ideal state of health, regardless of its nature or etiology' and as assessed by the respondent himself.

investigation, and the relevance, at this point in time, of any effort to understand individuals' choice of action in illness is clear from the previous chapter and from *Figure 2*. Several studies have been concerned with the broad outlines of the problem of how much ill health is seen in hospital, how much by general practitioners, and how much never reaches medical care,[6, 7] but they were not concerned with much detail of the population and of the diseases.[8,9] More detailed investigation began on a large scale with the United States National Health Survey[10] and the British Survey of Sickness.[11] Both of these studies pioneered questionnaires to establish morbidity in definite clinical terms. Further examples of national studies of this nature are given in Appendix I. Since these two surveys (with one interesting example[12]) there have been a series of investigations focusing in particular on the self-medication of morbidity. Jefferys *et al.* studied self-medication to establish whether it was being used as an alternative to consulting a general practitioner, and showed that it was not.[13] A later retrospective study in a general practice carried out by Kessel and Shepherd was concerned with consultation rates and self-medication, and came to conclusions similar to those of Jefferys.[14] Aspro-Nicholas[15] and Lader[16] have investigated self-medication too, but with greater emphasis on the types of medicine in use. More recently, Cargill[17] and the Office of Health Economics[18] have recommended the medical profession to review its attitudes to self-medication, with a view to becoming slightly more permissive. Cargill suggested, for example, that as an aid to easing the burden of work of a general practitioner some types of antibiotic should be made available as patent medicines.

The approaches used by social scientists to investigate what influences people's management of their complaints – and indeed of their health too – may be summarized as follows: is it largely something about the doctor, or about the individual himself, or about the nature of the illness, or is it some combination of these factors?

The first question – concerning the influence of the doctor and the relationship between the doctor and the patient – has received considerable attention, for example from Parsons,[19] Kosa,[20] Kadushin,[21] Cartwright,[22] and Balint.[23] Rosenblatt and Suchman have studied the attitudes towards and knowledge of health and illness in blue-collar workers, and conclude that they had a greater tendency to lack confidence in medical care than did white-collar and other professional workers, and thus since 'medical care will not become more parochial or less specialized' then 'if the social barriers are to be overcome, organizational means will have to be found to deal with these values on the part of the blue-collar workers'.[24] Other questions subsumed within this broad area include consideration of the effects of a previous unhappy experience in an episode of treatment, and fears of operations or investigation.

The second question – concerning the influence of the individual on his illness behaviour – has to be asked at several different levels. At its broadest, Dubos,[25] Titmuss,[26] Lewis,[27] and Susser and Watson,[28] among many others, have discussed variation and change in societal concepts of health and sickness. Other studies have investigated cross-cultural variations in definition and perception of sickness and health.[29, 30]

Societal attitudes and differing perceptions of health and illness may be seen, for example, in differences in attitudes to mental as opposed to physical illness. Thus the process of consulting medical care and having a complaint officially labelled may well constitute a difficult step. It can mean, as Parsons and others have suggested, that normal functions and duties may be relaxed while treatment for the illness is carried out, but it may also involve a degree of social stigma.[31, 32, 33] Choice of action for a complaint will therefore also involve considering the reactions of family, friends, workmates, and others to an official announcement of illness, and the material effects of such an announcement both on the individual himself and on his family and associates.[33, 34, 35, 36, 37, 38, 39, 40] Where prediction of behaviour at this individual level is concerned, the question is broadly this: is knowledge of an individual's social position a sufficiently powerful predictor of what we may expect of him in certain situations, or is the influence of an individual's interaction with others so strong that it is overridden? The first part of this question has been the one more commonly examined not only because of the relative ease of data-collection, but also because – as Zola has pointed out[41] – much illness is traditionally thought to be a direct and inevitable result of a particular social situation, namely poverty.

Finally there are a number of studies of the effect of the illness or complaint itself on its management by the sufferer. Different kinds of complaint will bring about different kinds of emotional response, and these, in turn, will be affected by the social environment. For example,

Rosenblatt and Suchman observe that for blue-collar workers 'symptoms which do not incapacitate are often ignored. For the white-collar group, illness will also relate to conditions which do not incapacitate but simply by their existence call for medical attention'.[42] Zbrowski[43] and Zola[44] have demonstrated cultural variations in reactions to complaints, and Mechanic and Volkart[45] have shown that persons with a high tendency to seek aid are significantly more likely to present 'routine' illness than persons with a low tendency. Cobb[46] has shown that differences in presenting patterns have made it look as if arthritis has been a disease predominantly of females. Gordon[47] has said that 'for all socio-economic groups, the major factor in defining someone as sick appears to be prognosis'. More recently, the results of a very broadly based and thorough study of this area have been published by Kalimo.[48]

It is helpful to quote Mechanic's summary to draw together some of the common difficulties experienced and the kinds of study reviewed in the foregoing selection and summary.

'Various studies of illness behaviour and medical care utilization in a variety of Western countries suggest that the actual use of medical services beyond a certain point has no very large relationship to the level of health. The medical care literature is primarily concerned with the practical issues surrounding utilization, delay in treatment and related matters. Much more serious, theoretical attention must be given . . . to the kinds of societal changes and new patterns of social relationships that produce high rates of utilization. Too few discussions in the utilization literature have struggled with the basic sociological dilemmas of health care: how can a society promote high levels of attention to symptoms and early symptom recognition without, in some measure, inducing hypochondriasis and how can medicine accommodate the large numbers of persons with psycho-social and psycho-somatic complaints when the most efficient bureaucratic form for scientific medicine is an alien one for dealing with such problems?'[49]

It is hoped, from research investigating these kinds of question, to piece together enough information to act as a predictive framework to assess how certain groups in particular communities will respond to specified complaints, and how they will respond to invitations for screening examinations, to prophylactic measures, and to health

14

education campaigns.[38, 50, 51, 52, 53, 54] The present study was begun in 1963, therefore, because we already believed it was time for us to begin to answer such questions as a step towards understanding the workings behind the epidemiologist's observation that 'needs have to be felt as such, perceived; then expressed in demand'.[55]

REFERENCES

1. MORRIS, J. N. (1967) *Uses of Epidemiology*, pp. 41–42. Livingstone, Edinburgh.
2. BUTTERFIELD, W. J. H. (1965) The orientation of the Consultant towards the New Approach to Public Health. *Public Health* **79** 218.
3. *The Times* (1969) Letter entitled Diagnosis Problem. 13 January, p. 7.
4. LOGAN, W. P. D., & BROOKE, E. H. (1957) The Survey of Sickness. *Stud. med. popul. Subj.* **12** HMSO, London.
5. HINKLE, L. E., REDMONT, R., PLUMMER, N., & WOLFF, H. G. (1960) An examination of the Relation between Symptoms, Disability and Serious Illness. *Amer. J. publ. Hlth* **50** 1327.
6. WHITE, K. L., WILLIAMS, T. F., & GREENBERG, B. G. (1961) The Ecology of Medical Care. *N. Eng. J. Med.* **265** 885.
7. HORDER, J., & HORDER, E. (1954) *The Practitioner* 173.
8. FROGGATT, P., & MERRETT, J. D. (1966) 'Proneness' of patients to consult their doctors. Paper to the Society for Social Medicine Conference, Edinburgh.
9. HOPE, K., & SKRIMSHIRE, A. (1968) Patient flows in the National Health Service. A Markov Analysis. Scottish Home and Health Department, Research and Intelligence Unit. Mimeo.
10. US National Health Survey. Public Health Service, Washington. Series A-1 (1958) Series B-1 (1957) et passim.
11. SLATER, P. (1946) *Survey of Sickness*. HMSO, London.
12. CLARK, A. J. (1938) *Patent Medicines*. Fact Monograph, No. 14, London.
13. JEFFERYS, M., BROTHERSTON, J. H. F., & CARTWRIGHT, A. (1960) Consumption of Medicines on a Working Class Housing Estate. *Brit. J. prev. soc. Med.* **14** 76.
14. KESSEL, N., & SHEPHERD, M. (1965) The Health and Attitudes of Persons who seldom consult a Doctor. *Medical Care* **3** 6.
15. ASPRO-NICHOLAS LTD. (1965) *Home Medication*. National Opinion Polls Ltd. NOP/1470 London.
16. LADER, S. (1965) A Survey of the Incidence of Self-Medication. *Practitioner* **194** 132.
17. CARGILL, D. (1967) Self-Treatment as an Alternative to Rationing Medical Care. *Lancet* **1** 1377.

18. OFFICE OF HEALTH ECONOMICS (1968) *Without Prescription*. Office of Health Economics, London.

19. PARSONS, T. (1965) *Social Structure and Personality*, pp. 112 and 257. Collier-Macmillan, London.

20. KOSA, J. *et al.* (1967) Medical Help and Maternal Nursing in Low Income Families. *Paediatrics* **5** 749.

21. KADUSHIN, C. (1962) Social Distance Between Client and Professional. *Amer. J. Sociol.* **67** 517.

22. CARTWRIGHT, A. (1967) *Patients and their Doctors*. Routledge and Kegan Paul, London.

23. BALINT, M. (1957) *The Doctor, his Patient and the Illness*. Pitman Medical Publication, Londons.

24. ROSENBLATT, D., & SUCHMAN, E. A. (1965) Blue Collar Attitudes and Information Towards Health and Illness, in *Blue Collar World* Shostak, A. B. and Gomberg. W. (eds), p. 324. Prentice-Hall, Englewood Cliffs.

25. DUBOS, R. (1960) *The Mirage of Health*. Allen and Unwin, London.

26. TITMUSS, R. M. (1958) *Essays on the Welfare State*. Allen and Unwin, London.

27. LEWIS, A. (1953) Health as a Social Concept. *Brit. J. Sociol.* **4** 109.

28. SUSSER, M. W., & WATSON, W. (1962) *Sociology in Medicine*. Oxford University Press, London.

29. LEIGHTON, A. H., & MURPHY, J. M. (1965) The Problem of Cultural Distortion. *Milbank Memorial Fund Quart.* **2** 189.

30. LAMBO, T. A. (1965) Contribution to discussion in *Milbank Memorial Fund Quart.* **2** 204.

31. PARSONS, T. (1964) *The Social System*. Chapter 1 – Social Structure and Dynamic Process: the Case of Modern Medical Practice, p. 428. Routledge and Kegan Paul, London.

32. MECHANIC, D. (1968) *Medical Sociology*. The Free Press, Glencoe.

33. MACLEAN, U. (1959) Community Attitudes to Mental Illness. *Brit. J. prev. soc. Med.* **23** 45.

34. KOOS, E. (1954) *The Health of Regionsville*. Columbia University Press, New York.

35. VINCENT, C. C. (1963) The Family in Health and Sickness. *Amer. Academ. pol. soc. Sci.* **346**. 109 in *Medicine & Society*, Clausen, J. A. & Strauss, R. (Eds.).

36. MARLOWE, D., & CROWNE, D. (1953) Social Desirability and Response to Perceived Situational Demands. *J. consult. Psychol.* **125** 109.

37. SAVIN, J. A. (1969) Social Behaviour and the Use of Medical Services. *Brit. J. prev. soc. Med.* **23** 53.

38. GRAY, R. M. KESLER, J. P., & MOODY, P. M. (1966) The Effects of Social Class and Friends' Expectations on Oral Polio Vaccination Participation. *Amer. J. publ Hlth* **12** 2028.

39. PHILLIPS, D. L. (1963) Rejection: a possible consequence of seeking help for mental disorders. *Amer. sociol. Rev.* **28** 963.

40. LEVINSON, D. J. MERRIFIELD, J., & BERG. K (1967) Becoming a Patient. *Arch. gen. Psych.* **17** 385.
41. ZOLA, I. K. (1965) Illness Behaviour of the Working Class: Implications and Recommendations, in *Blue-Collar World*, Shostak, A. B. and Gomberg, W. (Eds.) p. 350.
42. Op. cit. ROSENBLATT, D., & SUCHMAN, E. A. (1965) p. 341.
43. ZBROWSKI, M. (1958) Cultural Components in Responses to Pain, in Jaco. E. G. (ed) *Patients Physicians and Illnesses*, p. 256. The Free Press, Glencoe.
44. ZOLA I. K. (1965) Culture and Symptoms – an Analysis of Patients Presenting Complaints. *Amer. sociol. Rev.* **5** 615.
45. MECHANIC, D., & VOLKART, E. (1961) Stress, Illness Behaviour and the Sick Role. *Amer. sociol. Rev.* **26** 51.
46. COBB, S. (1963) Epidemiology of Rheumatoid Arthritis *Acad. Med. N.J. Bull.* **9** 52.
47. GORDON, G. A. (1966) *Role Theory and Illness – A Sociological Perspective.* p. 99. College and University Press, New Haven.
48. KALIMO, E. (1969) *Determinants of Medical Care Utilization.* National Pensions Institute, Finland. Series E:11/1969.
49. MECHANIC, D. (Unspecified date) The Sociology of Medicine: Viewpoints and Perspectives, p. 22. Mimeo.
50. BARSKY, P. N., & SAGEN, O. K. (1959) Motivation towards Health Examination. *Amer. J. Publ. Hlth* **49** 515.
51. HEASMAN, M. (1961) *Studies on Medical and Population Subjects.* **17** HMSO, London.
52. WAKEFIELD, J. (1963) *Cancer and Public Education.* Pitman Medical Publications, London.
53. UICC (1966) *Public Education about Cancer.* UICC, Geneva.
54. CRAVIOTO, J. (1960) Operation Zacatepec. *Int. J. Hlth Educ.* **3** 120
55. Op. cit. MORRIS, J. N. (1967) 82.

CHAPTER 3

The Study Area and its Population

INTRODUCTION

The study area has all the characteristics of old and well-established 'working-class' London, as opposed to those parts renowned for bright lights and entertainment, or the areas of constantly changing population, or the more peripheral newly developing areas. Bermondsey and Southwark appear very much to the fore in Mayhew's[1] list of districts where costermongers lived and worked.

Today, as in the late nineteenth century when Mayhew wrote, the area's character is largely determined by its proximity to the river, which forms the entire northern boundary, and by easy access to the City and to the commercial and industrial areas of east London. Consequently, it is dominated by concentrated traffic activity. Four trunk roads and two main railway lines cross the two boroughs from the suburbs and the country to reach the seven bridge-points forming the area's link with London north of the river. Four bridges and the Rotherhithe tunnel between them carry some 139,000 vehicles every twenty-four hours (1962 estimate)[2] and three bridges carry the rail traffic. The main-line terminal station at London Bridge, together with its adjacent Underground station, handled a *daily* total of 71,500 passengers in the study year (1963).

The busy nature of the two boroughs is reflected in the pattern of land-use. In Bermondsey more land is used by the railway and dock authorities than anyone else; ground used for housing came second, industry third, and roads fourth. In Southwark, while the greater land-usage is for housing, roads and industry are second and third. Southwark allocated proportionately more land for use as roads than was used in Bermondsey for housing.

The whole area is deficient in public open spaces. In 1945 the London County Council (as it then was) ruled that the ultimate standard of public open space per 1,000 persons was four acres and set an interim target of two and a half acres per 1,000 persons. In 1960, Bermondsey was still deficient even of the interim aim, with 1·7 acres per 1,000 persons, and Southwark had only 0·4 acres per 1,000 persons.

POPULATION STRUCTURE

For some considerable time the population of Bermondsey and Southwark has been falling steadily. Between 1931 and 1961 a drop of 48·8% per cent was registered, due for the greater part to war damage and slum clearance. The population, which had a high fertility rate in the late nineteenth and early twentieth centuries, is now ageing because of changes in the patterns of migration and mortality in more recent years.

TABLE 1

Age and sex structure of the sample compared
with three other populations

	(1961) Bermondsey & Southwark	(1961) Admin. County of London	(1961) England and Wales	(1963) Study Population
MALES				
20–39	19·8	19·9	18·6	16·6*
40–59	19·3	18·0	18·7	19·9
60 +	8·9	8·7	9·9	9·7
Total Males	48·0	46·6	47·2	46·2
FEMALES				
20–39	19·4	19·8	18·6	16·3*
40–59	18·4	19·2	19·7	20·7
60 +	14·2	14·3	14·6	16·8
Total Females	52·0	53·3	52·9	53·8
Grand Total (100%)	97,747	2,366,585	35,785,531	2,153

* Age-group 21–39 years.

19

Table 1 shows that the composition of the random sample used in the survey (drawn from the electoral register) was, in terms of age and sex, representative of the total population; there was, however, a tendency applicable to both males and females for the lower age-groups to be somewhat under-represented and the upper age-groups over-represented.

The marital status composition of the total population of Bermondsey and Southwark was almost exactly represented in the sample, with the exception of separated and divorced females, who were slightly over-represented.

In comparison with that of the Administrative County of London, and of England and Wales, the social-class structure of the two boroughs is weighted towards the lower end, and the sample population reflected this well.

The social-class structure of the sample consists, with the exception of 5·6 per cent, entirely of classes III, IV, and V, with 44 per cent of persons in classes IV and V.*

During 1963 in Bermondsey, the live birth-rate (per 1,000 population) was 17·5 and the corresponding figure for Southwark was 18·3. Also in 1963 the illegitimate birth-rate (expressed as a percentage of total live births) for both boroughs was approximately half that of London (14·2), standing at 7·0 for Bermondsey and 9·8 for Southwark. These figures represent quite a sharp rise in comparison, for example, with those of only five years earlier. Marriage rates for the same period have, on the other hand, dropped by about half, as a result of the migration of younger persons from the area, and the ageing population.

The sample over-represented small private households and quite seriously under-represented those in which six persons or more were living. Eleven (0·5 per cent) individuals interviewed were resident in households that contained more than ten people.

The appropriateness of the description 'well established' as applied to the area is made evident by details of where residents were born. Greater London was the birthplace of 84·8 per cent of the area's population, and the proportion of persons born outside the British Isles is among the lowest for any borough in London. Similarly, proportions of persons born in Scotland, Wales, and Ireland are

* We have used the classification of social class as defined by the Registrar General.[3]

low by average standards for London. The sample population is representative of the total population of the area, except in the case of residents who were born in countries outside Great Britain and the Commonwealth, which it under-represents, probably as a result of these persons not appearing on the electoral register.

EMPLOYMENT

Bermondsey and Southwark have as one of their most well-established industries the preparation and packaging of foodstuffs. This, together with the ease of access the area gives to the main centres of office accommodation where cleaners are needed daily, is the chief explanation for the high proportion of economically active women – one-third of all women, according to the Census data, and half of the study population. In the study population the most common occupations for women were office and general cleaner (21·4 per cent),* restaurant worker (16·9 per cent),* and office worker (16·1 per cent).* Men were chiefly employed in transport and communications (20·2 per cent),* and in the area's docks and warehouses. One man described his occupation as 'burglar'!

The most notable feature of the work of respondents was the high proportion who performed manual work (73·3 per cent of males), often with an equal division of time between outdoor and indoor activity. This may very well be in some part connected with the high proportion of rheumatic complaints, but it makes it surprising that there were so relatively few accidents reported.

HOUSING

No information concerning housing was collected from respondents in the course of the survey.

From the time of their industrialization until the 'Greenwood' Housing Act (1930),† Bermondsey and Southwark may by and large be said to have deserved their popular image as a slum, despite the good work of the famous Guy's prizewinner, Dr Alfred Salter, and others. But between 1931 and 1961, conditions improved enormously.

* As a percentage of all employed persons of the same sex.
† This Act provided subsidies for local authorities undertaking slum clearance and rehousing programmes.

The average number of persons per room dropped from 1·2 to 0·9, and the average number of persons resident per acre from 69·5 to 55·4. War damage (e.g. in Bermondsey 96 per cent of all dwellings were damaged) also helped to speed these changes.

In 1961, 43·7 per cent (21·2 per cent)* of all residents lived in accommodation rented from the local authority, 50·3 per cent (59·8 per cent)* rented their accommodation from private landlords, and only 1·7 per cent (15·6 per cent)* owned their dwelling. Most of the local-authority housing consisted of either recently built blocks of flats or late Georgian and nineteenth-century town houses entirely renovated. Special attention is now being given to the design of purpose-built accommodation for the aged and infirm. Privately rented dwellings are found either in large and often shabbily maintained tenement blocks, or in rows of terraced houses. During the year of the survey, 338 households (0·7 per cent of all households in the area) were registered as being in overcrowded circumstances, as defined by the 1957 Housing Act.

GENERAL STATE OF HEALTH

Table 2 gives some idea of how much the general state of health of the area's total population had improved over the period of forty years between 1923 and 1963, the year of the survey. The borough councils and medical officers of health had been especially careful to act on Dr Salter's advice:

'Add to good houses, wider streets, more open spaces, open-air schools, pure milk and a general raising of the standard of living, and tuberculosis will disappear like typhus and the Black Death.'[4]

Bermondsey, in particular, was not only unusual in its far-reaching plans for conversion to a 'garden city', but also for its original efforts at health education and the control of disease. In 1923 a mobile film unit was introduced which would stop in a suitably busy thoroughfare to instruct passers-by in the care of their teeth and to show such works as *Where There's Life There's Soap*. The Solarium and the spacious public baths were opened in 1926 and 1927

---

* Figures in parenthesis give 1961 figures for the Administrative County of London; others refer to Bermondsey and Southwark.

TABLE 2

General and selected* mortality rates for Bermondsey only, for 1923 and 1963, all ages

Rate	1923	1963
Crude mortality rate	12·1	12·6
Infant mortality rate	76·0	15·8
Deaths from respiratory disease†	33·2	11·6
Deaths from measles	0·9	—

* The mortality rates are expressed as per 1,000 live births/deaths, and the remainder as percentages of all deaths for that year.
† This term includes deaths from influenza, pulmonary tuberculosis, bronchitis, pneumonia, and the category 'other respiratory disease' specified in the contemporary MOH annual reports which are the source for this table.

respectively, and these events received publicity on a national scale for their high standards made available to the 'working man'.

A present-day well-documented health hazard is air pollution, and the local health authorities are much concerned with it. In April 1963 deposited matter collected during the month on one site represented 40·2 tons per square mile and in July at another site the comparable figure was 8·3 tons. Other measurements for 1963 fall within the range 8–40 tons.

Such high levels of pollution should be set against the area's high rate of deaths from lung cancer and bronchitis, which between 1949 and 1960 were both consistently higher than the overall rates for England and Wales. On the other hand, over the same period, with the exception of 1949, death-rates from cardiovascular disease in Bermondsey were every year less than those for England and Wales.

MEDICAL-CARE FACILITIES

1. *Hospitals*

As *Map 1* shows, Bermondsey and Southwark are well provided with hospitals within easy reach. At the time of the survey, however, the distinction between teaching and district general hospitals seemed well pronounced. We found[5] that, between 1950 and 1960, Guy's was providing for 24 per cent of the local bed needs and 40 per cent of all local outpatient needs. In 1965, this situation was changed with the

Map 1 Hospitals in south-east London

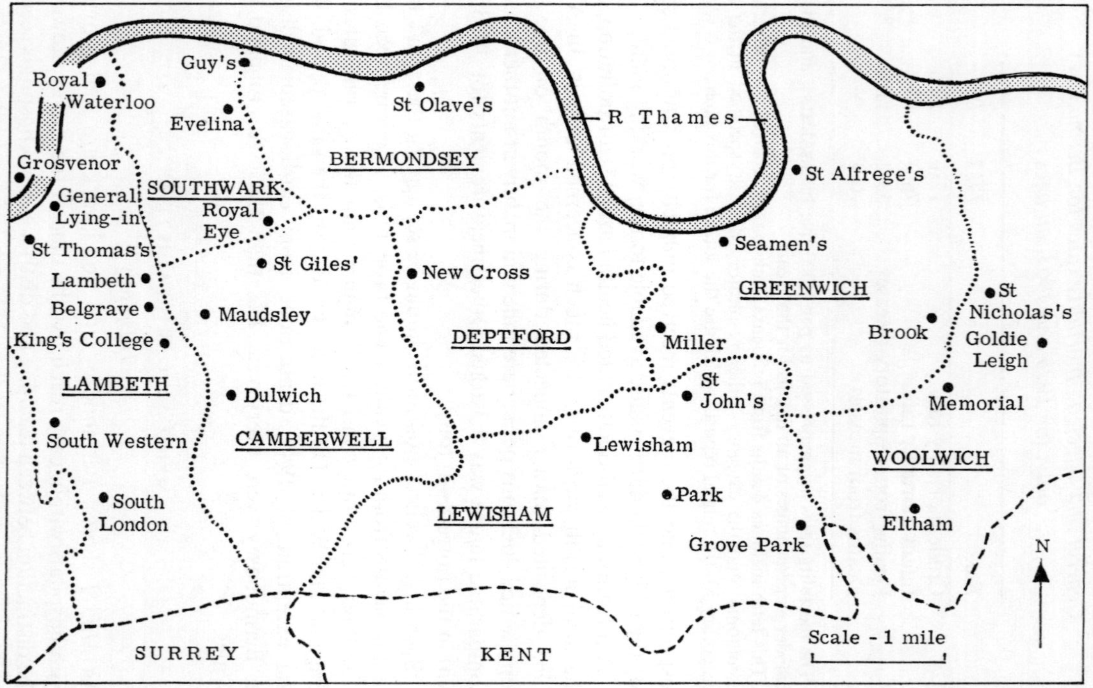

introduction of the Guy's Hospital Group, which has in its jurisdiction Guy's, the Evelina, St Olave's, and New Cross hospitals. Thus the responsibilities of the teaching hospital were extended. Some indication of the distribution of catchment areas before the formation of the new group may be gathered from *Map 2*, which shows the distribution of general practice premises around Guy's Hospital. The highly localized allegiance to St Olave's (coping with 42 per cent of Bermondsey admissions) and to the Lambeth hospitals (coping with 26 per cent of Southwark admissions) is clear, and is a phenomenon that grew as the neighbouring teaching hospitals became increasingly specialized (30 per cent of Guy's beds were, in 1962, occupied by local residents). Undoubtedly the new group will do something to redress this situation.

2. *General Practitioners*

At the time of the survey, 74 doctors were working in 46 practices in Bermondsey and Southwark, an overall distribution of 2,133 persons per doctor. *Map 2* shows the distribution of these practices throughout the district and *Table 3* shows the structure of practices.

TABLE 3

The structure of general practices
in Bermondsey and Southwark (1963)

Type of Practice	%
Single-handed	60·9
Partnership of 2	23·9
Group of 3	8·7
Group of 4	6·5
Total (100%)	46

Although almost all the general practitioners were exceptions to the overall rule for Central London, in that they had practised in the district for quite some time, very few of them actually lived in Bermondsey or Southwark. In 1963 their mean age was 50·3 years. Relationships between hospitals and general practices in the area, which have been shown to be not ideal,[6] are now improving, particularly as a result of hospital case conferences and other meetings and the introduction at Guy's of open-access diagnostic facilities.

25

Map 2 Distribution of general practitioners in Bermondsey and Southwark showing outpatient departments most used in 1963

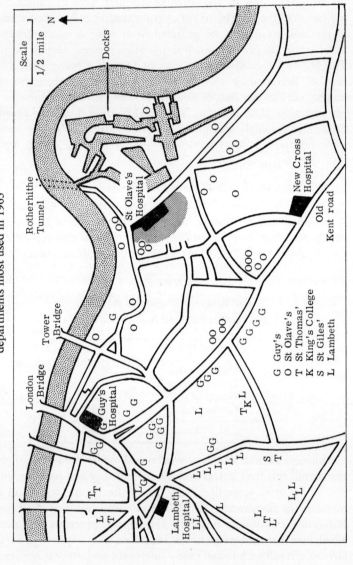

3. *Local Authority Care*

Map 3 shows the distribution of the main services provided by the local authorities, as well as some other facilities. In 1963, both Bermondsey and Southwark were notable for their provision for the welfare of the elderly. Day centres, chiropody, laundry, meals on wheels, workshop, and holiday home services were all coping with an increasing number each year.

At the time of the study many of the services shown in *Map 3* were under the administration of the London County Council Health Division 8. Since this included an area considerably greater than just Bermondsey and Southwark it is impossible to give estimates of staffing. It is clear, however, both from *Map 3* and from personal experience, that the area is well provided for.

CONCLUSION

In this chapter we have described the key aspects of our study population and its environment, and made some comparisons with other populations. As a sample of the total population of Bermondsey and Southwark it is sufficiently representative, but these two boroughs are in some ways rather different from England and Wales as a whole. We need to be explicit as to how these differences will hinder us in extrapolating from our data to the whole population.

The most obvious area of difference is that of social class. Bermondsey and Southwark have a predominantly low social-class structure as compared with England and Wales. Economic activity is also different. Women work, especially in part-time jobs, much more commonly than do women in the total England and Wales population. The environment of the study area is unusual, even by other urban area standards, because of its very high density of resident population and its concentrated traffic activity. Whereas the average number of residents per acre in the total Greater London conurbation in 1961 was 17·7, and the highest figure outside the immediate area of London was for Salford (29·6), the figures for the study area had by 1963 *dropped* from previous levels to 43·5 persons per acre in Bermondsey and 76·3 in Southwark. How will these differences affect any desire to apply our conclusions to the national population?

Map 3 The main local-authority health and welfare centres in Bermondsey and Southwark at the time of the study

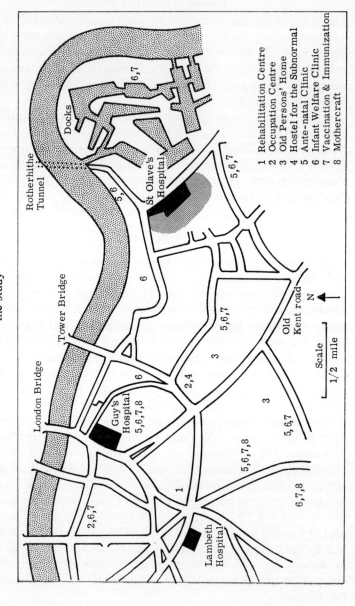

1 Rehabilitation Centre
2 Occupation Centre
3 Old Persons' Home
4 Hostel for the Subnormal
5 Ante-natal Clinic
6 Infant Welfare Clinic
7 Vaccination & Immunization
8 Mothercraft

First, the social-class difference will be a hindrance. There is no way of avoiding this, especially since nationally there is a tendency towards an overall rise in social class. Marsh[7] shows that between 1931 and 1961 the proportion of all occupied and retired males in England and Wales in social classes I and II rose from 15 per cent to 19 per cent, and that in classes IV and V dropped from 36 per cent to 30 per cent.

Second, in economic activity, Bermondsey and Southwark are certainly different from England and Wales, but here the difference is forward-looking, since the Census data show that the national trend is, as the base-line of positions open to women broadens, towards this difference. The proportion of all women aged 15 years and over who were economically active in 1951 was 34·8 per cent and this had risen, according to the 1961 10 per cent sample census, to 37·7 per cent.

Third, the high density of resident population and the concentration of traffic. The difference between Bermondsey and Southwark and the national (England and Wales) average is anticipatory. The 1961 Census showed that 80 per cent of the total England and Wales population lived in urban areas, and that the number of towns with a population of over 50,000 had risen steadily, so that 53·3 per cent of the total population then lived in such towns. Even the populations of all the conurbations had increased by proportions in the range 0·15 per cent to 4·89 per cent between 1931 and 1961, with the exception of Greater London, where a drop of 1·98 per cent was recorded. Along with this there is undoubtedly an increasing amount and concentration of traffic activity, and, as far as trends may be said to be discernible in such a wide field, there does seem to be a growing desire on the part of planners for higher-density (in all its many senses) urban residence.

In addition to these trends *Table 4* shows the similarity in changes in population age-structure between England and Wales, on the one hand, and Bermondsey and Southwark. Thus, with the exception of social class, the points of difference between the study area and the national average are not necessarily to be seen as a hindrance but more as an aid to extrapolation and future prediction. Here, of course, we are open in particular to two criticisms. First, that we have chosen only a limited number of variables on which to base our comparison. And, second, that although trends do seem inclined

TABLE 4

Age distribution of Bermondsey and Southwark, and England and Wales compared for a 50-year period
England and Wales figures in brackets, and totals in thousands
Compiled from Census data

Age-groups	1911	1921	1931	1951	1961
0–24	51·6 (48·7)	49·5 (45·3)	46·1 (41·2)	35·5 (35·0)	36·0 (36·1)
25–49	34·3 (35·3)	33·4 (35·7)	33·9 (36·1)	38·8 (37·1)	34·7 (33·3)
50–74	13·3 (14·6)	15·6 (17·3)	18·5 (20·6)	22·4 (24·3)	25·1 (26·3)
75–84	0·8 (1·3)	1·5 (1·5)	1·4 (1·8)	2·9 (3·1)	3·6 (3·6)
85 +	0·1 (0·2)	0·1 (0·2)	0·2 (0·2)	0·4 (0·5)	0·6 (0·7)
Total (= 100%)	317,810 (36,070·5)	303,856 (37,886·7)	283,237 (39,952·4)	157,861 (43,757·8)	138,109 (46,104·8)

towards some important aspects of Bermondsey and Southwark's present state, conditions (such as high-density traffic routes near residential areas) will be improved.

In answer to the first criticism, we have chosen those variables which may both be collected at household interviews and be comparable with data collected by the Registrar General.

While admitting the truth of the second criticism, it must be seen against two other important points. First, that for the great majority of persons improvements are only rarely and then usually gradually becoming part of the trends outlined above. Second, that whatever the changes in environment there seems no reason to suppose that the tendency for the 'diseases of civilization'[8] (and also see Chapter 1) to increase will change in the face of the growth of many factors associated with civilization and the development of urban life.

REFERENCES

1. MAYHEW, H. (1851) *London Labour and the London Poor*, 2 vols. G. Woodfall and Son, London.
2. MINISTRY OF TRANSPORT (1963) Personal communication.
3. GENERAL REGISTER OFFICE (1966) *Classification of Occupations*. HMSO, London.
4. BROCKWAY, F. (1951) Quote from Salter in *Bermondsey Story*, p. 97. Allen and Unwin, London.

5. BUTTERFIELD, W. J. H., BLANEY, R., WADSWORTH, M. E. J. (1966)
A London Teaching Hospital, in *Problems and Progress in Medical
Care*, p. 128. Oxford University Press, London.
6. ACHESON, R. M., BARKER, D. J. P., & BUTTERFIELD, W. J. H., (1962)
How General Practitioners Use Out Patient Services in Two
London Boroughs. *Brit. med. J.* **2** 1315.
7. MARSH, D. C. (1967) *The Changing Social Structure of England and
Wales, 1871–1961*, p. 133. Routledge and Kegan Paul, London.
8. For example YUDKIN, J. (1967) Evolutionary and Dietary Changes in
Carbohydrates. *Amer. J. clin. Nutn.* **20** 108; and SUKHATME
P. V. (1967) FAO Rome. Personal communication.

CHAPTER 4

General Review of the Findings

Each interview began with the question 'Would you say that your state of health during the last fourteen days was perfect, good, fair, or poor?' Almost one-third (35 per cent) of respondents assessed their state of health as 'perfect', 34 per cent felt in 'good' health, 21 per cent said that their health was 'fair', and 10 per cent felt in 'poor' health. The greater proportion of those who felt in fair or poor health were significantly more likely to have been widowed or separated or divorced.*

Of the total number of respondents (2,153 = 100 per cent), no health complaints were reported by 105 (4·9 per cent). Both the pilot study for this survey and the Peckham Health Centre study[1] found that 12 per cent of their sample populations had no complaints. The explanation of this difference lies in the construction of the present questionnaire (see Appendix I). The method of cross-checking information by the use of correlated checklists not only of symptoms but also of medicines, action taken, and chronic diseases and impairments has here ensured close accuracy of data concerning action taken, and also accumulated extensive details of symptom states.

No action was taken by 405 (18·8 per cent) respondents for complaints reported, and the remaining 1,643 (76·3 per cent) persons had taken some kind of action for their complaints.

THE COMPLAINTS REPORTED

Table 5 gives details of all complaints reported at interviews, whether in answer to a question or offered spontaneously, and ranks them in order of frequency. It is important to emphasize that this table is concerned with *complaints*, and that the International Standard Classification Code (ISC code) categories have been used only as a convenient form for grouping.

* Chi-square significant at the 0·05 level.

TABLE 5

All reported active complaints by ISC (4-digit) classification, in rank order

ISC classification	No.	%
Respiratory system	2,397	25·7
Mental, psychoneurotic, etc., disorders	1,968	21·1
Bones and organs of movement	1,433	15·4
Digestive system	1,012	10·9
Nervous system and sense organs	719	7·7
Skin and cellular tissue	502	5·4
Circulatory system	393	4·2
Accidents	316	3·4
Ill-defined conditions	212	2·3
Genito-urinary system	208	2·2
Congenital malformation	71	0·8
Infective and parasitic disease	60	0·6
Pregnancy and complications	13	0·1
Allergic, endocrine, metabolic, and nutritional disease	10	0·1
Neoplastic disease	1	0·01
Total	9,315	100·0

In view of the nature of the area from which the study population was drawn, both geographical and demographic factors may well have contributed significantly to make respiratory disorder the most common complaint. Studies of populations consulting general practitioners have found very similar rank-ordering of frequency of complaints, and where definitions of categories allow comparison there is a quantative similarity also. For example, disorder of the respiratory system was reported by 26 per cent of both the present study's population and a general-practice population.[2] Two other groups are comparable. Of our population, 8 per cent complained of disorder of the nervous system and sense organs, as did 8 per cent of the same general-practice population, and 11 per cent of both populations reported complaints of the digestive system. Of course, the different methods of selecting the two populations and of categorizing complaints reduce the value of these comparisons.

We shall now examine the five most common complaints, namely those of respiratory, mental, rheumatic, digestive, and skin disorders, in relation to the main social factors collected about each respondent.

More complaints were reported by women than by men. Where age was concerned, only respiratory complaints showed almost no fluctuation between ten-year age-groups. Rheumatic complaints increased with increasing age (mean 52·3 years, SD 16·4); mental disorders were commonest in the 40–49 year age-group, then in the 21–29 and the 30–39 year groups, and then decreased as age increased (mean 49·3 years, SD 16·1); digestive complaints were commonest in the 30–39 year group (mean 43·9 years, SD 27·3), and skin complaints were most often reported by those between the ages of 21 and 39 years (mean 47·5 years, SD 6·0).

Mental and rheumatic disorders both showed increased proportions of complaints from the widowed and the separated and divorced, and whereas there was very little variation in the proportions of complaints reported by those suffering respiratory complaints, digestive disorders were commonest among the single (13 per cent of all complaints from single persons), then among the married and the separated and divorced (in each case 12 per cent), and least from widows (10 per cent). Complaints of skin disorder were greatest from the single (10 per cent of all complaints from the single), next from married persons (8 per cent), then from the widowed (7 per cent), and finally from the separated and divorced (5 per cent). The commonest types of complaint by single, widowed, and separated and divorced persons were mental disorders, and the commonest by the married were rheumatic disorders.

Reporting by social classes I and II was proportionately greater than by any other class in respiratory and rheumatic complaints, 34 per cent of all complaints by these classes was of respiratory complaints and 41 per cent of rheumatic disorder. Reporting of mental disorder, of digestive complaints, and of skin complaints increased with descending social class.

Employed persons reported proportionately the most only in the case of skin complaints. Respiratory and rheumatic disorders were most often reported by the retired, mental disorders by housewives, and digestive disorders by the unemployed.

There were no notable trends in reporting in relation to household size, except in the case of digestive complaints, which increased with increasing household size.

Table 6 shows the ten most commonly reported chronic complaints (see Appendix I). Of the total of 603 conditions reported as 'active'

TABLE 6

The ten most commonly reported chronic* complaints, according to states of activity and arranged in rank order

Condition reported	Active in last 14 days	Still active but not in last 14 days	Cleared up by operation	Cleared up by itself or with treatment	Total (100%)
Bronchitis	12·8	24·5	—	62·7	482
Rheumatism	36·8	37·9	—	25·3	383
Haemorrhoids	12·9	28·3	8·2	50·6	233
Varicose veins	25·7	60·0	6·7	7·7	222
Fibrositis	13·3	23·5	—	63·3	196
Lumbago	8·2	22·4	—	69·4	183
Hypertension	17·7	27·0	—	55·3	141
Mental or nervous disorder	20·0	46·9	—	33·1	130
Migraine	16·8	46·4	—	36·8	125
Hernia and rupture	8·5	11·3	67·0	13·2	106
All chronic complaints	19·8	29·7	8·2	42·4	3,017

* See Appendix I for definition of 'chronic'.

nt the time of interview 71 per cent had been medically diagnosed. Respondents were asked whether they had ever suffered from any of the chronic complaints on the checklist (see Appendix I) and all reports were categorized, if not currently active, as cleared up by operation, or of their own accord, or with treatment. All active complaints of chronic illness are included in tables of complaints unless otherwise specified.

WHO MADE THE DIAGNOSIS

For each of their complaints, respondents were asked who had, at any time and not just during the previous fourteen days, originally made the diagnosis. The replies, grouped according to whether the diagnosis was made by a medically qualified person or not, and by disease group, are given in *Table 7*. This table requires caution in interpretation. It is made up on the one hand of respondents' reports of diagnoses made by a medically qualified person at some time in the past, but not necessarily in the preceding fourteen days. On the other hand these reports are compared with respondents' own grouping of their disorders. Thus figures showing medical diagnoses are, in accordance with the accuracy of the respondent's memory and the doctor's clear, full, and accurate explanation, fitted within the ISC groups, whereas figures showing non-medically qualified diagnoses are likely to be much less well fitted to the classifications. For example, a complaint reported as backache, and caused perhaps by renal disorder or gynaecological disease, could here be classed as a disorder of the bones and organs of movement. Within these limitations the important figures in this table are the percentages of complaints medically diagnosed, and it is interesting to note the frequency with which the respondents acted as diagnosticians.

TABLE 7

Complaints according to who had originally made the diagnosis

| Rank order | ISC disease category | Who diagnosed | | Total |
		Doctor	Respondent	(100%)
1	Respiratory system	37·0	63·0	2,397
2	Mental, psychoneurotic, etc.	19·6	80·4	1,968
3	Bones and organs of movement	39·2	60·8	1,433
4	Digestive system	22·7	77·3	1,012
5	Nervous system and sense organs	40·9	59·1	719
6	Skin and cellular tissue	27·3	72·7	502
7	Circulatory system	42·0	58·0	393
8	Accidents	22·0	78·0	316
9	Symptoms and senility NEC*	27·4	72·6	212
10	Genito-urinary system	23·6	76·4	208
11	Congenital malformation	85·9	14·1	71
12	Infective and parasitic disease	58·3	41·7	60
13	Pregnancy and complications	100·0	—	13
14	Allergic and endocrine disease	70·0	30·0	10
15	Neoplastic disease	100·0	—	1
	Total	32·0	68·0	9,315

* NEC means throughout 'not elsewhere classified'.

The social factors collected about each respondent were checked against the author of the diagnosis for each of the five commonest complaints to see if any of them significantly differentiated those whose complaints had been diagnosed by a doctor from those who

36

had made their own diagnosis. Sex was important in mental, digestive, and rheumatic disorders. In each of these cases significantly more females than males had consulted a doctor,* and the greatest difference was for digestive disorder.

Age was of significant importance in each of the five groups of complaints. In rheumatic, digestive, and respiratory complaints the percentages of persons consulting the doctor rose with increasing age, and in each case chi-square was significant at the 0·001 level. In complaints of mental disorder, in which of all of these five groups the doctor was least likely to have made the diagnosis, respondents most often consulted in the age-group 30–39 years, and then 50–59 years and over 70 years (chi-square significant at the 0·05 level). Skin complaints were most often diagnosed by a doctor in the 40–49 year group, followed by the 60–69 year group and the 21–29 year group (chi-square significant at the 0·01 level).

Marital status was of significance for four groups, but not in the case of digestive disorder. In both respiratory disorder (chi-square significant at the 0·05 level) and mental disorder (chi-square significant at the 0·01 level) divorcees most often consulted, and in rheumatic complaints and those of skin troubles (for both, chi-square significant at the 0·01 level) widows most often consulted.

Where social class was concerned, four groups of disorders were significantly associated with whether or not a doctor had been consulted, the exception being skin disorder. Respiratory and mental disorders were more often diagnosed by a doctor when suffered by persons in social classes I and II (chi-square in each case significant at the 0·001 level), but for digestive and rheumatic disorders the lower the social class the greater the likelihood of medical consultation (chi-square significant respectively at the 0·05 and 0·02 levels).

Employment status was of significance for every group of complaints, and in all cases except that of skin disorder the unemployed and the retired were the most likely to have consulted the doctor (in each case chi-square significant at the 0·001 level, except for digestive disorder where it was at the 0·2 level). Skin complaints were most often taken to the doctor by housewives, and this was significant at the 0·05 level.

Household size was of importance in mental disorder (0·01 level),

* Chi-square significant for digestive and mental disorders at the 0·001 level, and for rheumatic complaints at the 0·05 level.

where the peak of medical consultations was reached in households of four, and in respiratory complaints (also significant at the 0·01 level) in households of two and of four persons. Frequency of having consulted a doctor with rheumatic complaints was greatest in households of six and more, and then in households of one and two (0·001 level).

In addition to this descriptive work, we also used our main variables describing each respondent in a further analysis. The variables used were age, sex, social class, employment status, marital status, household size, and the total number of all complaints reported by the respondent concerned. Using these, a multiple regression analysis was carried out to discover whether any of these seven variables accounted for some part of the difference between those persons who had at some time taken the complaint studied to a doctor and those who had never done so. Results are given in each of the following five chapters which describe the five most common complaints and how respondents managed them, in some detail.

ACTION TAKEN FOR THESE COMPLAINTS

Table 8A shows the types of action taken during the fourteen days before interview, with the exception of medicine-taking, and *Table 8B* shows when the general practitioner was last consulted. Eighteen respondents (0·8 per cent) were not registered with a doctor. 'Lay advice' in *Table 8A* includes the person who had been to an osteopath and the person who had consulted a faith-healer.

The national average for the ratio of surgery consultations to home visits by general practitioners is approximately 2 to 1, and another study[3] found a 3 to 2 ratio. The finding of 10 to 1 in this study, although not strictly comparable, is of some interest, and will have been largely affected, we think, by the large number of surgery premises close together in this area (see *Map 2* in Chapter 3), and by the likelihood that, since very few of the general practitioners lived in the area, they would have discouraged home visiting.

Of the total study population 3 per cent (69 persons) – and twice as many women as men – had received certificates for sickness absence during this period before the interview. Of these, two-thirds were National Insurance Certificates, as compared with the finding of one-third in another study.[3]

TABLE 8A

Action taken in the fourteen days before interview,
for all complaints

Medical measures		No.	As a percentage of all respondents
Visited a family doctor		254	11·8
Hospital outpatient treatment		56	2·6
Visited a GP dentist		51	2·4
Visited by a family doctor		39	1·8
Hospital inpatient		10	0·5
Saw a doctor at work		6	0·3
Visited hospital casualty		5	0·2
Visited hospital dentist		3	0·1
Visited optician		6	0·3
	Total	430	20·0
Local authority measures			
Help from borough council*		42	2·0†
Seen by doctor in LCC clinic		38	1·8
Visited chiropodist		24	1·1
Visited an ante-natal clinic		17	0·8
Visited by a health visitor		7	0·3
	Total	128	6·0
Other measures			
Days off work/housework		174	8·1
Days in bed		104	4·8
Asked advice of a chemist		26	1·2
Asked lay advice		19	0·9
	Total	323	15·0

* Meals on wheels, appliances, home help, and home laundry.
† 15·7% of respondents were aged over 60 years.

A wide range of medicines was in use. The 486 medicines are shown in *Table 9*, which also gives the percentage of respondents taking them and the number of different preparations and brands in each group. Of the medicines identified, analgesics were taken by a large proportion of respondents (38 per cent), followed by skin medicines, lower-respiratory medicines and antacids. The category of 85 'other

TABLE 8B

When the general practitioner was last consulted

Period during which last consultation occurred	Percentage
0–13 days	13·6
14 days–5 months, 3 weeks	25·8
6 months–11 months, 3 weeks	15·4
1 year—	25·5
4 years—	5·6
10 years +	2·8
Never	9·4
Unknown	1·9
Total (100%)	2,153

TABLE 9

Medicines and appliances, by the percentage of all respondents who had used them in the previous fourteen days, for all sources of prescription

Type of medicine	Percentage of respondents (100% = 2,153)	No. of brands* in each group
Analgesics	38·1	22 (4·5%)
Other medicines and means†	27·1	85 (17·5)
Skin medicines	20·4	70 (14·4)
Appliances	15·3	37 (7·6)
Other and unspecified medicines	13·4	Unknown
Lower-respiratory medicines	13·1	37 (7·6)
Antacids	12·1	22 (4·5)
Counter-irritants	10·8	34 (7·0)
Tonics and vitamins	10·8	42 (8·6)
Salts	10·7	9 (1·9)
Laxatives and purgatives	9·1	24 (4·9)
Medicines usually medically prescribed	6·3	27 (5·6)
Upper-respiratory medicines	4·8	24 (4·9)
Ear and eye medicines	4·2	16 (3·3)
Sedatives	3·8	6 (1·2)
Antibiotics and other anti-infective agents	3·2	12 (2·5)
Heart, urinary, and kidney medicines	2·6	7 (1·4)
Other gastro-intestinal medicines	1·5	12 (2·5)
Total		486 (100·0)

* For example, each manufacturer's brand of aspirin was considered separately.
† See Appendix II.

40

medicines and means' used by 583 (27 per cent) respondents ranged over a vast spectrum from herbal preparations to ear trumpets, and from the use of copper bracelets as a prophylactic measure against arthritis to self-cauterization of a laceration.

In identifying medicines, interviewers noted brand names, and failing this the intended action, or the part of the body concerned. If none of these was possible then the medicine was recorded as 'other and unspecified', and of these 88 per cent had been medically prescribed.

For every medicine prescribed by a doctor, two were taken either on the respondent's own initiative or on that of some other lay person, or, very rarely, in any event during the fourteen days before interview, on the advice of a chemist (see *Table 8A*). As the number of complaints rose, there was a corresponding rise in the amount of medically prescribed medicine taken and a fall in lay prescription. This trend was quite consistent, from the 8 per cent of medically prescribed medicines taken by those persons reporting one complaint to the 33 per cent taken by those reporting more than ten complaints.

As compared with our finding of 33 per cent of medicines being medically prescribed, a market research group[4] found 23 per cent of medicines were medically prescribed. The difference in these figures may well be accounted for by our use of a much more detailed questionnaire that was able to discover medicines taken regularly over a long period for chronic disease (for example, insulin for diabetes) which a questionnaire specifically seeking information about self-medication might miss.

TABLE 10

Mean number of medicines used, by age and sex

		10-year age-groups					
		21–29	30–39	40–49	50–59	70–69	70 +
Mean no.	Males	1·5	1·6	1·7	2·1	2·5	2·3
of medicines	Females	1·9	2·2	2·3	2·2	2·3	2·6

Table 10 shows the mean number of medicines used in the fourteen-day pre-interview period, according to the age and sex of the users. Females took more medicines than males. The mean number of

medicines used by males was 1·9 and by females 2·2. The narrowing of this difference between the sexes after 50 years of age is in agreement with the finding of a similar study carried out on a broadly comparable population.[5] Females took more than average quantities of the following medicines, the figure in parenthesis being the difference between the sexes in amounts taken:

Laxatives and purgatives	(24·2%)
Other gastro-intestinal medicines	(43·8%)
Tonics and vitamin preparations	(24·4%)
Ear and eye medicines	(20·8%)
Antibiotics	(21·0%)
Heart, urinary, and kidney medicines	(21·4%)
Other and unspecified medicines	(23·6%)

Of our population, 19 per cent of persons were taking some kind of prophylactic medicine or action at the time of interview and this was, in the case of the 14 per cent of persons doing so on their own initiative, most often salts of some kind, orange juice and vitamin preparations, exercise, or aspirin.

ATTRIBUTED CAUSES

We divided reports of attributed causes into those diagnosed by the doctor and those made by the respondent himself or by some other lay person, and then each of these was subdivided into three types of cause, namely physical, psychological, and environmental. The findings are shown below.

Diagnoses made by the doctor		*Diagnoses made by a lay person*
Physical	86·7%	62·1%
Psychological	8·9%	7·7%
Environmental	4·4%	30·2%
Total (=100%)	2,981	6,334

It was not entirely surprising to find that lay persons more commonly attributed their complaints to environmental causes, but the similarity in the psychological causes was unexpected. Details of causes attributed to each of the five most common complaints are discussed in Chapters 5–9.

REFERENCES

1. PEARSE, I. H. & CROCKER, L.H., (1943) *The Peckham Experiment.* Allen & Unwin, London.
2. GENERAL REGISTER OFFICE (1962) Studies on Medical & Population Subjects. No. 14: *Morbidity Statistics from General Practice.* HMSO, London.
3. SCOTT, R., ANDERSON, J. A. D., & CARTWRIGHT, ANN (1960) Just What the Doctor Ordered. *Brit. med. J.* **2** 293.
4. NATIONAL OPINION POLLS LTD., for Aspro-Nicholas (1965) *Home Medication.* 2 NOP/1470.
5. JEFFERYS, MARGOT, BROTHERSTON, J. H. F., & CARTWRIGHT, ANN (1960) Consumption of Medicines on a Working Class Housing Estate. *Brit. J. prev. soc. Med.* **14** 72.

CHAPTER 5

Respiratory Complaints

Respiratory disorders made up the most common cause of complaint and accounted for one in four (27 per cent) of all complaints. According to Fry this should not be surprising in view of the ecology of the area concerned. He notes[1] a tendency for such infection to be more prevalent in the lower social groups, and goes on to point out his finding that 'the incidence of most respiratory infections was higher in urban areas . . . The explanations usually offered are the effects of atmospheric pollution and the opportunities for cross-infection from overcrowding at home, at work and in travel.'[2] Chapter 3 has shown how the people from the area concerned in this study fulfil all the qualifications that have seemed to many researchers contributory to a high prevalence of respiratory disorders.

The commonness of this group of complaints in all sorts of populations and environments in England and Wales is well demonstrated by three of the standard measures of the effect of illness on the community. The first of these is that of medical prescribing statistics. These show that more than one-tenth of prescribing expenditure is for chronic bronchitis.[3] The second is the number of working-days lost as a result of the condition concerned. In the year 1960–1961, for example, 21·7 per cent of all working-days lost were due to chronic bronchitis and acute respiratory disease.[4] The final measurement is that of total National Health Service expenditure on the condition. Respiratory disease is the third most costly set of illnesses in these terms, accounting for 8·3 per cent of the total National Health Service expenditure.[5] Furthermore, one study in general practice showed that 23 per cent of all consultations during the study period were for respiratory disease.[6]

One of the greatest difficulties encountered in an attempted measurement of the effects of respiratory disease is that of defining the disease itself. Fry, for example, says that there are 'more than

44

one hundred synonyms for infections of the lungs',[7] and the problem was thoroughly discussed at an international conference on Comparability in Epidemiological Studies.[8] In the present study, however, the nature of the investigation (an assessment of action taken for complaints) minimized the problem of definition. As indicated in Appendix I, questions specifically designed to discover details of respiratory complaints were either exact copies of, or were based on, well-validated questions previously used in morbidity studies.

WHO REPORTED THESE COMPLAINTS

Table 11 shows complaints of respiratory disorder reported in this study. A little more than one-quarter (29 per cent) of these data were volunteered by respondents without the use of a question, and these are contained in the categories 'coughs and colds' and 'influenza'. As well as these complaints which were active at the time of the interview some chronic respiratory illness in various stages of inactivity was also reported (*Table 12*).

TABLE 11

Grouped respiratory complaints relating to a 14-day period

Complaint	No.	%
Colds and coughs	661	36·6
Coughing spit or phlegm	365	20·0
Regularly coughed spit or phlegm	335	18·4
Shortness of breath worse than other people	207	11·4
Severe chest pain or discomfort	106	5·8
Bronchitis	64	3·5
Frequent sinus trouble	37	2·0
Influenza	35	1·9
Asthma	10	0·01
Coughing up blood	2	0·001
Total	1,822	100·0

Although for respiratory complaints as a whole there was more reporting by women than by men, the opposite was true in the case of coughing spit and phlegm and of upper-respiratory complaints.

Whereas complaints of lower respiratory disease increased with age

45

TABLE 12

Activity states of reported chronic respiratory complaints

Complaint	Cleared up by operation	Cleared up by itself or with treatment	Active at present	Still active but no symptoms in last 14 days	Total (=100%)
Asthma	—	38·1	23·8	38·1	42
Bronchitis	—	62·7	12·8	24·5	482
Sinus trouble	13·8	4·6	42·5	39·1	87

(the sharpest increases were in the case of coughing spit and phlegm and of shortness of breath), upper-respiratory complaints decreased with age from 21 per cent of those aged 21–29 years, to 14 per cent of those aged 60 years and over.

There were no notable trends in reporting in relation to social class.

Where employment status was concerned, complaints of shortness of breath, severe chest pain, and coughing spit and phlegm were most commonly reported by the unemployed (36·7 per cent of the unemployed), followed by the retired (26 per cent) and housewives (14 per cent), and finally by those employed both full time and part time (13 per cent). All remaining complaints varied very little as between employment statuses, and most were reported by the unemployed (12·8 per cent of those unemployed), and least by the retired (12 per cent).

Married persons reported most upper-respiratory complaints (17 per cent of all married persons) and separated and divorced persons most low respiratory complaints (20 per cent).

WHO MADE THE DIAGNOSIS

The mean number of complaints that had originally (i.e. not necessarily in the previous fourteen days) been seen and diagnosed by a doctor amounted to one-third of the total number of complaints (37 per cent). There was, however, a wide variation in this rate as between complaints, as is shown in *Table 13*.

There were a few significant associations between these complaints and whether or not they had ever been taken to a doctor. Upper-respiratory complaints were much more often taken to medical care by the unemployed than by any other employment group (86 per cent of those unemployed, or 24 per cent of those employed – chi square significant at the 0·01 level). Lower-respiratory complaints – with the exception of severe chest pain and shortness of breath – were significantly more often taken to a doctor as the individual's total number of complaints rose. In this case chi-square was significant at the 0·01 level. Social class was only of significant importance in complaints of shortness of breath, and respondents of social classes I and II were more likely to have consulted a doctor (chi-square significant at the 0·01 level). Complaints of coughing spit and phlegm were significantly most commonly taken to the doctor by those aged over 50 years (28 per cent, chi-square significant at the 0·02 level).

TABLE 13

Respiratory complaints according to who originally made the diagnosis

Complaint	Who diagnosed		Total ($=100\%$)
	Doctor	Other	
Coughing up blood	—	100·0	2
Shortness of breath	27·8	72·2	207
Severe chest pain or discomfort	25·7	74·3	106
Coughing spit or phlegm	17·3	82·7	365
Has coughed spit and phlegm*	21·5	78·5	575
Regularly coughs spit and phlegm	23·7	76·3	335
Coughs and colds	35·5	64·5	661
Influenza	37·1	62·9	35
Asthma	70·0	30·0	10
Bronchitis	67·4	32·6	64
Frequent sinus trouble	43·8	56·3	37
Total	37·0	63·0	2397

* But not in the last 14 days.

Multiple regression analysis showed that in the case of upper-respiratory disorders the difference between those ever consulting a doctor and those never doing so was best explained by unemployment, which accounted for 4·6 per cent of the difference, and, together with sex, for 5·7 per cent. All variables together accounted for 9·8 per cent of the difference. In lower-respiratory disease the difference was best explained by the total number of all complaints reported, and all variables considered together accounted for 14 per cent of the difference. In complaints of coughing spit and phlegm the difference was most significantly explained by the total number of all complaints reported (3·8 per cent of the difference), and all variables accounted for 5 per cent of the difference. In complaints of shortness of breath social class explained 3·2 per cent of the difference, being of single marital status 1·5 per cent, and all variables considered together 7·8 per cent of the difference.

ACTION TAKEN

Table 14 summarizes the measures respondents had taken for these complaints during the previous fourteen days. Of all measures taken, medical care was the most common, and within this category complaints were mostly taken to the general practitioner (65 complaints), but in 19 cases the general practitioner made a home visit. Thus, for every complaint of respiratory disease involving a visit by the general practitioner, he saw three in the surgery. The next commonest measure was to go to the outpatients department (5 complaints) or a local-authority clinic (4 complaints). Two of those complaining had been seen in hospital, two by a doctor at work, and one had been visited by a health visitor.

Thirty-four per cent of these complaints were being medicated during the fourteen days before interview; *Table 15* gives details.

Upper-respiratory complaints were the most commonly medicated – medically or lay – (70 per cent of all upper-respiratory diseases), followed by lower-respiratory complaints (38 per cent). Lower-respiratory complaints, with the exception of coughing spit and phlegm, severe chest pain, and shortness of breath, were the most commonly medically medicated (37 per cent of these complaints), and upper-respiratory complaints (50 per cent) the most often lay-medicated. Of all complaints reported during this study, respiratory complaints were most often being treated by lay persons with several medicines at the same time (4·3 per cent of these complaints), and most often treated with several lay-prescribed medicines as well as medically prescribed medicines (3·2 per cent of these complaints).

For self-medication respondents chiefly put their faith in analgesics (mainly aspirin), patent respiratory medicines, antacids and tonics and vitamin preparations, as well as in a number of unorthodox medicines.* (See also Appendix II, *Table A*.)

* For example, alcohol, honey preparations, lemon-juice, breathing exercises.

TABLE 14

Action taken for respiratory complaints over a period of 14 days

Action	No. of complaints	
Sought medical care	98	(4·1%)
Stayed away from work	73	(3·0%)
Went to bed	25	(1·0%)
Asked non-medical advice	14	(0·6%)
No action	2,187	(91·2%)
Total	2,397	(100·0%)

TABLE 15

Prescription of medicine for respiratory complaints

Medicine group	Who prescribed		Total persons medicating (=100%)
	Doctor	Self	
Analgesics	6·7	93·3	150
Antacids	10·8	89·2	37
Laxatives and purgatives	100·0		4
Salts	—	100·0	8
Other gastro-intestinal medicine	50·0	50·0	2
Counter-irritants	50·0	50·0	8
Upper-respiratory medicine	35·0	65·0	80
Lower-respiratory medicine	42·6	57·4	275
Tonics and vitamin preparations	17·3	82·7	15
Skin medicines	100·0	—	8
Ear and eye medicines	—	100·0	1
Antibiotics and other anti-infectives	90·0	10·0	30
Heart, urinary, and kidney medicines	100·0	—	8
Sedatives	100·0	—	3
Medicines usually medically prescribed	88·9	11·1	27
Other and unspecified medicines	82·5	17·5	80
Appliances	—	100·0	2
Other medicines and measures	15·4	84·6	78
Total (=100%)	38·1	61·9	816

ATTRIBUTED CAUSES

Doctors were most often said to have diagnosed these complaints as being of physical origin (96 per cent of those disorders which were diagnosed by the doctor), whereas respondents themselves felt that 70 per cent of the complaints they had diagnosed were the result of physical causes. Both doctors and lay persons were reported as attributing 1 per cent of these complaints to psychological causes, and environmental factors were said by doctors to have accounted for 3 per cent of these complaints and by lay persons for 30 per cent. The most common of these was tobacco-smoking, which accounted for more than half, followed by the outside environment and the weather (for example, wet and cold weather, and traffic fumes and other atmospheric pollution), and work activity and environment. Worry and personal stress were usually said to be the cause of lay-diagnosed complaints of shortness of breath and severe chest pain.

SUMMARY

Upper-respiratory complaints and those of coughing spit and phlegm were reported more often by males than by females, and all other complaints were more often reported by females. With the exception of upper-respiratory complaints, where reporting decreased with age, for all other complaints it increased with age. Complaints of shortness of breath, severe chest pain, and coughing spit and phlegm were proportionately more often reported by those not in employment. There were no notable trends in reporting in relation to social class.

Of all these complaints 37 per cent had originally been diagnosed by a doctor. The unemployed significantly more often consulted a doctor in the case of upper-respiratory complaints, those in social classes I and II in complaints of shortness of breath, those aged over 50 years in complaints of coughing spit and phlegm, and those with a larger number of complaints in the case of all other respiratory disorder. Multiple regression analysis accounted for 9·6 per cent of the difference between those consulting a doctor and those not doing so in the case of upper-respiratory complaints, 14 per cent of the difference in lower-respiratory disorders, 5 per cent in complaints of coughing spit and phlegm, and 7·8 per cent in complaints of shortness of breath.

In the fourteen days before interview doctors had been consulted about 3 per cent of these complaints, 34 per cent of complaints were being medicated, and a little more than one-third of medicines in use had been medically prescribed.

Environmental factors were ten times more frequently cited as the cause of complaints by lay persons than by medical practitioners in making a diagnosis.

REFERENCES

1. FRY, J. (1962) *Morbidity Statistics from General Practice*, p. 19. HMSO, London.
2. FRY, J. op. cit. 32.
3. OFFICE OF HEALTH ECONOMICS (1964) *The Cost of Medical Care*, p. 20.
4. MORRIS, J. N. (1964) *Uses of Epidemiology*, p. 34. Livingstone, Edinburgh.
5. OFFICE OF HEALTH ECONOMICS. Op. cit. 16.
6. FRY, J. op. cit. 15.
7. FRY, J. op. cit. 16.
8. MILBANK MEMORIAL FUND (1965). Comparability in International Epidemiology. *Milbank Memorial Fund Quarterly*, **43** No. 2 Part 2, 77–126, et passim.

CHAPTER 6

Complaints of Tiredness, Worry, Nervousness, and Headache

One of the fields of medical care that has changed most drastically, even since the second world war, is that of mental illness. Some indication of the size of this, 'the most serious medical problem', has been given as follows:

> An investigation of the incidence of psychological illness in a British general practice showed that about 10 per cent of adult patients on a doctor's list will receive treatment in any one year for an unequivocally psychiatric complaint. The inclusion of patients with symptoms for which no physical cause can be found and those considered to suffer from 'psychosomatic' or 'stress' disorders raised this proportion to about 50 per cent. Only a small proportion of these patients are referred by their doctors to psychiatric clinics but, even so, patients with neurotic and personality disorders constitute some two-thirds of all the patients seen at clinics of this type.[1]

Increasing awareness of mental illness as a problem badly in need of a solution, together with an increasing range of medicines available for the support and active therapy of the mentally sick, and wider recognition of mental illness, are all making considerable demands on the services providing medical care.

In economic terms the burden of mental illness on the National Health Service bill is currently estimated to be in the order of £140,000,000 annually. Of all disorders in 1961–1962 (the year before the fieldwork for the present study) mental health required the greatest expenditure, using almost twice as much as any other disorder.[2]

The effect on hospitals might be summarized by saying that an increasing number of people are now able to be admitted as inpatients for a greater number of shorter periods.

Local health authorities are more and more concerned with mental health. Between 1961 and 1964 the number of persons in England and Wales receiving mental health care from this source rose by 78 per cent.[3]

Figures for the load of mental illness in general practice as a whole are not available, but it is at least certain that the family doctor is actively concerned at some stage with many of those receiving hospital and local-authority care. It has been estimated that 14·3 per cent of all morbidity experience in an 'average British practice of 2,500 persons' may be ascribed to 'emotional disorders'.[4]

Perhaps the most striking description of the situation was made by the Office of Health Economics. 'For every patient in hospital suffering from mental illness there are two in the community: the local authorities look after only one tenth of this number' and 'bear the greatest burden in the public care of the mentally subnormal'.[5]

In the present study there were 1,968 complaints of worry, nervousness, tiredness, and headaches, and these represented 21 per cent of all complaints, the second largest group. They were reported by 1,830 persons. Details of these complaints are given in *Table 16*.

TABLE 16

Grouped complaints of tiredness, worry, nervousness, and headache relating to a 14-day period

Complaint	No.	%
Headache NEC	409	20·8
Tiredness	390	19·8
Very run down all the time	371	18·9
Difficulty in sleeping	289	14·7
Worry or depression worse than other people	184	9·3
Worry NEC	158	8·0
Severe headache	106	5·4
Mental and nervous disorders	61	3·1
Total	1,968	100·0

As well as those complaints active at the time of interview, 69 persons reported previous chronic episodes of 'mental and nervous disorder', which for the greater part (43) had already been cleared up with treatment, and the rest (26) were no longer troublesome at the time of interview. Most (60) of all these 69 complaints had been diagnosed by a doctor.

WHO REPORTED THESE COMPLAINTS

For each of these complaints there was more reporting by females than by males, the latter reporting 43 per cent of complaints, and the former 58 per cent. The greatest differences were in the case of worry or 'depression felt to be worse than average', severe headaches, and mental and nervous disorders.

Whereas complaints of worry and depression and of difficulty with sleeping rose with increasing age (to 27 per cent and 26 per cent of those aged over 60 years) those of headaches fall with age (from 35 per cent at 21–29 years), and complaints of feeling run-down remained quite steady at 27 per cent, with the exception of a peak of 35 per cent in the 40–49 year age-group. This peak was accounted for by reporting from female respondents.

Those who were widowed, separated, and divorced most often reported each of these kinds of complaints, whereas married and single persons had lower rates of reporting, except in the case of headaches, which were complained of by 29 per cent of married persons.

Reporting by social class declined with descending social class in complaints of difficulty with sleeping. Worry and depression was least reported by social class III (14 per cent of this class) and most by social classes I and II (19 per cent).

For each of these complaints reporting was at its lowest from those employed, and highest from the unemployed. Differences of only 5 per cent in proportions of housewives and retired persons reporting were the same for all complaints with the exception of headache, reported by 31 per cent of housewives as opposed to 18 per cent of retired persons.

WHO MADE THE DIAGNOSIS

Table 17 shows who had originally (that is not necessarily in the previous fourteen days) diagnosed the complaints. Complaints least

TABLE 17

Complaints of tiredness, etc., according to who originally made the diagnosis

Complaint	Medically diagnosed	Non-medically diagnosed	Total (= 100%)
Headache NEC	25·4	74·6	409
Tiredness	19·0	81·0	390
Very run down all the time	13·5	86·5	371
Difficulty in sleeping	7·3	92·7	289
Worry or depression worse than others	17·4	82·6	184
Worry NEC	32·1	67·9	158
Severe headache	15·1	84·9	106
Mental and nervous disorder	59·1	40·9	61
Total	19·6	80·4	1,968

often taken to the doctor were those of severe headache, feeling very run-down, and difficulty with sleeping. Only a quarter of headaches not specified as severe had been seen by a doctor. One-third of the complaints of worry and depression had been diagnosed medically, as had more than a half (59 per cent) of mental disorder.

For some of these complaints there were certain personal attributes and facts about respondents' social situations that were associated with whether the complaints have ever been diagnosed by a doctor. For difficulty with sleeping and worry and depression, however, there were no significant correlations. Persons complaining of headaches were significantly more likely to have gone to a doctor if they were retired (27 per cent of retired persons) or housewives (25 per cent) or unemployed (13 per cent). The chi-square test was significant at the 0·001 level. Only 11 per cent of employed persons had consulted a doctor about headaches.

There were also significant differences between persons who did or did not consult a doctor and who complained of feeling very run-down and tired. Again, the unemployed (44 per cent of all those unemployed), the retired (34 per cent), and housewives (30 per cent) more often consulted than the employed (27 per cent); chi-square was significant at the 0·001 level. Also in the case of complaints of being very run-down and tired, the widowed and the divorced were the most likely to have consulted medical care, and so

55

were females rather than males, and those living alone rather than those living with others. In the case of each of these, chi-square was significant at the 0·01 level.

Multiple regression analysis showed that in complaints of tiredness the variable that contributed most to our understanding of the difference between those who had gone to the doctor with this complaint and those who had not was the total number of complaints reported, which accounted for 3 per cent of the difference between the two sorts of respondent. When the variables widowhood, unemployment, and age were added we could account for 6·1 per cent of this difference. When all seven variables used in the multiple regression analysis are considered together, we could explain 10·1 per cent of the difference. In the case of headache the most important single variable was the status of housewife, which accounted for 2·1 per cent of the difference, and the inclusion of age and widowhood raised this figure to 3·9 per cent. All variables taken together explained 5·2 per cent of the difference between the two groups. One other complaint was of some small significance in this analysis – difficulty with sleeping. Although no one variable contributed very much, consideration of all the variables explained 5·0 per cent of the difference between the two groups of respondents.

ACTION TAKEN

Only 73 complaints (3·7 per cent of all complaints in this group) had been referred to a medical-care agency in the fourteen-day period leading up to the interview, and details are given in *Table 18*. The most common medical measure taken was to consult a family doctor at his surgery. This outweighed having a doctor come to his home to visit the patient by 12 to 1. Nine persons had been to a hospital out-patient department in the fourteen-day period; two had been in-patients. The local authority had been actively concerned with three cases, one had been seen by a doctor at work, two by opticians, and two by dentists. (See also Appendix II, *Table B*.)

Whereas only 4 per cent of these complaints had been taken to medical care, 592 (30 per cent) had been in some way medicated during the same period. Lay medication outweighed medical prescription by two to one, as is shown in *Table 19*. By far the most common medicines used were analgesics, and of these 88 per cent were non-

TABLE 18

Action taken for complaints of tiredness, etc. over a period of 14 days

Action	No.	%	As a percentage of all these complaints
Sought medical care	73	56·6	3·7
Stayed away from work	34	26·4	1·7
Went to bed	16	12·4	0·8
Asked non-medical advice	6	4·7	0·3
Total	129	100·0	6·5

TABLE 19

Percentage of complaints of tiredness, etc., for which medicines were taken, and who prescribed the medicine

Complaint	Percentage of complaints medicated		Total no. of complaints
	Doctor	*Other*	
Headache	10 0	43 8	403
Tiredness	16·4	14·6	390
Very run down	6·5	7·5	371
Difficulty sleeping	5·9	10·4	289
Worry and depression	4·3	1·1	184
Worry NEC	31·6	15·2	158
Severe headache	5·7	44·3	106
Mental and nervous disorder	14·8	9·8	61
Total	219 (11·1)	373 (19·0)	1,968 (100·0)

medically prescribed. Other medicines largely lay-prescribed were antacids, laxatives, salts, and respiratory preparations. Headaches, and specifically severe headaches, were complaints most often lay-medicated, for the most part with analgesics. Lay medication for severe headaches outweighed medical prescription by eight to one, and for other headaches by four to one.

ATTRIBUTED CAUSES

Doctors were said to have attributed 59 per cent of these complaints about which they had been consulted at some stage to the result of a physical disorder, 37 per cent to a psychological problem, and 4 per cent to some environmental cause. Respondents said that of the complaints that they had themselves diagnosed 22 per cent were due to a psychological problem, 26 per cent to environmental factors, and 52 per cent to a physical disorder. Environmental causes were most often work activity and environment, home environment, and personal stress and worry.

SUMMARY

These complaints were notable because, although they showed a tendency to be more commonly reported by social classes I and II, social class was of no significance in differentiating those persons who sought medical care from those who had not. Of all those complaining 20 per cent had at some time been seen by a doctor. The doctor was significantly more likely to have been consulted by respondents who were not employed, by females, by those living alone, by the widowed, and by the divorced. However, only a small percentage of the difference between those seeking medical advice and those not doing so could be accounted for by our variables, even when all seven were taken into consideration, in the case of three types of complaint, namely tiredness (10·1 per cent), headache (5·2 per cent), and difficulty with sleeping (5 per cent).

Although 4 per cent of all these complaints had been referred to doctors during the fourteen days before interview, 30 per cent were being in some way medicated, and a little more than one-third of the medicines had been medically prescribed. Whereas doctors were reported to have attributed the majority of the complaints that they had diagnosed to some physical disorder, respondents were much more inclined to cite environmental factors as causative of lay-diagnosed complaints.

REFERENCES

1. JONES, H. GWYNNE (1966) Neuroses, Extreme Anxiety and Irrational Behaviour. *Progress in Mental Health*, p. 8. Office of Health Economics.
2. Op. cit. OFFICE OF HEALTH ECONOMICS (1966) *Progress in Mental Health*, p. 28.
3. Op. cit. OFFICE OF HEALTH ECONOMICS (1966) p. 39.
4. FRY, J. (1964) General Practice Tomorrow. *Brit. Med. J.* **2** 1065.
5. Op. cit. OFFICE OF HEALTH ECONOMICS. (1966) p. 40.

CHAPTER 7

Rheumatic Complaints

'Rheumatological research, for so long the Cinderella of medicine . . .'[1] is a remark that applies in many ways as much to everyday management of these conditions as to research.

The high prevalence of these disorders can hardly be doubted. One report[2] gave a list of fourteen 'rheumatic' conditions (including rheumatoid and unspecified arthritis, but excluding gout, rheumatic fever, and prolapse of the intervertebral disc) with their consultation rates as calculated from a study in general practice, and the overall consulting rate was 88·9 patients per 1,000 at risk. Another study[3] in an 'average' general practice ranked the rates of presentation of disorders, and the combination of acute back pain and rheumatoid arthritis made up the fifth commonest group, namely 3·6 per cent of all presenting symptoms.

High prevalence is not limited solely to Britain. In the United States these diseases are said to be the commonest cause of chronic illness, and rank second in causing 'temporary or permanent disability'.[4] An estimated one in twenty persons in the United States suffers 'some form of rheumatic disease', and it is thus 'more common than the total number of cases of tuberculosis, diabetes, cancer and heart disease combined'.[4]

In the year 1960–1961, two years before the present fieldwork was carried out, the estimate of weekdays lost from work by insured men in Britain was 17 million days for 'rheumatism, arthritis, sciatica, etc.'.[5] This was the third most incapacitating disease according to this particular index.

It has also been estimated that disease of the bones and organs of movement (following the International Standard Classification Code) was the tenth most expensive group of illnesses in terms of National Health Service expenditure in England and Wales in the year 1961–1962.[6]

TABLE 20

Grouped rheumatic complaints relating to a 14-day period

Complaint	No.	%
Low back pain	797	55·6
Bad limb pain	196	13·7
Bad joint pain	165	11·5
Rheumatism	141	9·8
Bone and joint disorder NEC	48	3·3
Other arthritis	31	2·2
Fibrositis	26	1·8
Lumbago	15	1·0
Slipped disc	7	0·5
Rheumatoid arthritis	7	0·5
Total	1,433	100·0

While it is evident that insufficient details are given here of the composition of each of these indices, it is enough to show that these conditions are very commonly presented to medical care, and it would thus be reasonable to expect a high rate of complaint from a random sample of a community.

Altogether there was a total of 1,433 complaints in this category, and they formed the third largest group, 15 per cent of all complaints reported. Details are given in *Table 20*.

It was not by any means unexpected to find these complaints so commonly occurring in view of the ecology of the community. It has a low social-class structure, a high proportion of manual workers, a lot of inferior and damp housing, and it is sited on old marshland surrounding the docks. For the same reasons it was not surprising to find low back pain the commonest cause of complaint, followed by joint pain and then limb pain.

Table 21 (p. 62) shows how many respondents felt a chronic complaint was latent. In all cases, except for the two types of arthritis, reports of latent disease exceeded the number of complaints active at the time of interview.

WHO REPORTED THESE COMPLAINTS*

Whereas complaints of pain in the joints and pain in the limbs rose

* In this section all complaints were grouped under three headings, namely pain in the joints, pain in the limbs, and low back pain.

TABLE 21

Activity states of reported chronic rheumatic complaints

Complaint	Cleared up by operation	Cleared up by itself or with treatment	Active at present	Still active but no symptoms in last 14 days	Total (= 100%)
Rheumatism	—	25·3	36·8	37·9	383
Fibrositis	—	63·3	13·3	23·5	196
Lumbago	—	69·4	8·2	22·4	183
Other arthritis	—	32·5	38·8	28·8	80
Slipped disc	3·6	42·9	25·0	28·6	28
Rheumatoid arthritis	—	30·0	70·0	—	10

steadily with age (the former from 24 per cent of the 21–29 age-group to 53 per cent of those over 60 years, and the latter from 19 per cent of the youngest group to 42 per cent in the older group), low back pain was most often reported in the years 30–49 (25 per cent of these persons) and those aged over 70 years (24 per cent). Women reported more complaints than men, except in the case of complaints reported specifically as lumbago.

Widows and divorcees more often complained of limb pain (41 per cent of these respondents) and of joint pain (47 per cent) than did married or single persons, and in the case of low back pain there was very little variation in reporting according to marital status.

Employed persons, whether in full-time or part-time work, reported fewer complaints than those in other employment groups; complaints were commonest from the retired.

Reporting of limb pain and joint pain increased with descending social class (limb pain 28 per cent of social classes I and II, and 33 per cent of class V, and joint pain 35 per cent of classes I and II, and 41 per cent of class V. Low back pain showed a similar trend, but least frequent reporting was in social class III (14 per cent).

WHO MADE THE DIAGNOSIS

Table 22 shows these complaints according to who originally had made the diagnosis.

Employment status and social class were most often of significance

TABLE 22

Rheumatic complaints according to who originally made the diagnosis

| Complaint | Who diagnosed | | Total |
	Doctor	Other	($= 100\%$)
Low back pain	40·5	59·5	797
Bad limb pain	21·0	79·0	196
Bad joint pain	25·5	74·5	165
Rheumatism	49·6	50·4	141
Bone and joint disorder NEC	43·7	56·3	48
Other arthritis	74·2	25·8	31
Fibrositis	84·6	15·4	26
Lumbago	66·7	33·3	15
Slipped disc	100·0	—	7
Rheumatoid arthritis	71·4	28·6	7
Total	39·2	60·8	1,433

in distinguishing those who had sought medical care and those who had not done so. When all these complaints were put into three groups – joint pain, limb pain, and low back pain – those who, in each group, had been to a doctor with these complaints were significantly more often not employed and unemployed (for joint pain and limb pain chi-square is significant at the 0·05 level, and for limb pain at the 0·001 level).

Low back pain was significantly more often taken to the doctor by those in social classes III and IV (chi-square significant at the 0·001 level), and joint pain more often by social classes I and II (chi-square significant at the 0·05 level).

Limb pain was significantly more often taken to the doctor as age increased (chi-square significant at the 0·001 level), and by those who lived alone (57 per cent of those living alone) or those who lived with one other person (52 per cent). In this case the chi-square test was significant at the 0·01 level.

Joint pain that had been medically diagnosed was significantly associated with an increase in the total number of complaints suffered (chi-square significant at the 0·02 level).

Multiple regression analysis showed that the difference between those ever demanding medical care and those never doing so with complaints of low back pain was best explained by age, which accounted for 1 per cent of the difference, and by social class, which covered a further 1·6 per cent. All variables together explained 6·0 per cent of the difference. In complaints of joint pain the total number of all complaints reported accounted for 1·8 per cent of the difference, and retirement a further 1·4 per cent. All variables together accounted for 5·9 per cent of the difference. Age was the most important source of explanation of the difference between the two groups in the case of limb pain, and this variable explained 2·5 per cent. All variables considered together accounted for 5·4 per cent of the difference.

TABLE 23

Action taken for rheumatic complaints over a period of 14 days

Action	No.	%	As a percentage of all these complaints
Sought medical care	77	67·0	5·4
Stayed away from work	23	20·0	1·6
Went to bed	14	12·2	1·0
Asked non-medical advice	1	0·8	0·1
Total	115	100·0	8·1

ACTION TAKEN

Table 23 summarizes measures taken for this group of complaints during the fourteen days before interview.

Of the 73 persons who had received medical care in the previous fourteen days, more than half (42) had consulted a general practitioner at his surgery, and six had been visited in their homes by a doctor. One had consulted a doctor at work, and 23 had been seen at hospitals. The local authority was providing some form of help for one person; one person was going to a day hospital and four to chiropodists. Only a small number had stayed away from work (23), and 14 people had gone to bed as a result of their complaint.

Of all these complaints 46 per cent were receiving some sort of medication during the fourteen days before the interview. *Table 24* shows the percentages of each complaint medicated, according to who had prescribed the medicines. Thirty-one different kinds of medicines were identifiable.

The most commonly used lay-prescribed medicines were counter-irritants, followed by analgesics and then various sorts of appliances, such as thermogen wool.

Several lay-prescribed medications were being used simultaneously by fifty persons, and sixty-two persons were using both medically prescribed and lay-prescribed medicines at the same time. (See also Appendix II, *Table C.*)

TABLE 24

Percentage of rheumatic complaints for which medicines were taken, and who prescribed them

Complaint	Percentage of complaints medicated Doctor	Other	Total no. of complaints
Low back pain	18·3	37·9	797
Bad limb pain	5·1	12·2	196
Bad joint pain	7·9	9·1	165
Rheumatism	24·8	32·6	141
Bone and joint disease NEC	29·2	35·4	48
Other arthritis	9·7	16·1	31
Fibrositis	11·5	11·5	26
Lumbago	60·0	20·0	15
Slipped disc	28·6	14·3	7
Rheumatoid arthritis	—	28·6	7
Total	235 (16·4%)	427 (29·8%)	1,433 (100%)

ATTRIBUTED CAUSES

Following almost exactly the same pattern as for respiratory disorders, medical opinion was reported to have attributed 95 per cent of these complaints to physical causes, 1 per cent to psychological causes, and 4 per cent to environmental causes. Respondents themselves ascribed 68 per cent of lay-diagnosed complaints to physical causes, 30 per cent to environmental causes, and 0·3 per cent to psychological causes. Work, housework, and the weather (in that order) were most commonly given as environmental causes.

SUMMARY

Although the incidence of all these complaints rose with age, low back pain was also common in the 30–49 year age-group. Employed persons complained less often than others, and reporting was higher in the lower social classes. Of these complaints, 39 per cent had originally been diagnosed by a doctor. The employed were less likely to have sought medical advice for these disorders than were persons in any other employment state. Proportionately more of those in social classes I and II consulted a doctor about joint pain, and proportionately more of those in social classes III and IV did so about low back pain. Limb pain taken to the doctor was associated with increasing age and with living alone or with one other person. During the fourteen days before interview, 5 per cent of these complaints had been attended to by a doctor and 46 per cent were being medicated.

Lay persons were much more likely in their diagnoses to attribute complaints to environmental causes than were doctors who, it was reported, ascribed physical causes to 95 per cent of disorders that had been referred to them.

REFERENCES

1. COPEMAN, W. S. C. (1966) In a speech at the opening of the Mathilda and Terence Kennedy Institute of Rheumatology, October 6th. Quoted in *The Times*, 7 October.
2. WALFORD, P. A. (1962) *Morbidity Statistics from General Practice* III, p. 77. HMSO, London.
3. FRY, J. (1964) General Practice Tomorrow. *Brit. med. J.* 2, 1065.
4. HOLLANDER, J. L. (ed.) (1953) *Arthritis and Allied Conditions*. Kimpton, London. Quotation of official statistics, p. 19.
5. MORRIS, J. N. (1964) *Uses of Epidemiology*, p. 34. Livingstone, Edinburgh.
6. OFFICE OF HEALTH ECONOMICS (1964) *The Costs of Medical Care*, Table A.8.

CHAPTER 8

Digestive Complaints

Although not among the most expensive of disorders (ranking sixth in the Office of Health Economics classification of National Health Service expenditure), digestive diseases were found in two studies in general practices to form the third largest group of complaints presented.[1, 2] Thus these general practitioners probably saw two or three patients each working-day who were suffering from such disorders. As they point out, however, 'this does not mean . . . that diseases of the digestive tract occupied third place in the amount of work done', although 'in many cases . . . a long course of treatment may be required'.[1] Patients who had circulatory disease were seen in the study just quoted almost twice as frequently as were those with digestive disease, 'and so, if the number of consultations per patient is taken to represent the amount of work involved, "diseases of the digestive tract" come to occupy fourth place'.[1]

The 1,012 complaints reported in the present study made up the fourth most common reason for complaint, and 11 per cent of all complaints. *Table 25* gives details of this group, and *Table 26* shows the chronic complaints reported.

WHO REPORTED THESE COMPLAINTS

There was more reporting by females than by males for all digestive complaints with the exception of obesity, blood in the bowel motions, and diarrhoea, where in each case there was a very small excess of reporting by males.

Complaints of a very poor appetite rose with age, those of stomach upset and indigestion (and this includes heartburn, nausea, vomiting, abdominal pain, and all kinds of ulcers, as shown in *Table 25*) reached peaks in the age-groups 30–39 years and over 70 years. Complaints of diarrhoea reached a peak in the 30–49 age-group and weight change in the 30–39 age-group. Complaints of indigestion and

TABLE 25

Grouped digestive complaints relating to a 14-day period

Complaint	No.	%
Indigestion, heartburn, nausea, vomiting	374	37·0
Stomach upset, gastro-enteritis	236	23·3
Very poor appetite	173	17·1
Diarrhoea	71	7·0
Big loss in weight	53	5·2
Dental disorder	52	5·1
Blood in bowel motions	24	2·4
Obesity	10	1·0
Hernia or rupture	9	0·9
Stomach, peptic, or duodenal ulcer	7	0·7
Gall-bladder or liver trouble	3	0·3
Total	1,012	100·0

TABLE 26

Activity states of reported chronic digestive complaints

Complaint	Cleared up by operation	Cleared up by itself or with treatment	Active at present	Still active but no symptoms in last 14 days	Total (= 100%)
Hernia or rupture	67·0	13·2	8·5	11·3	106
Stomach, peptic, or duodenal ulcer	40·8	33·8	9·9	15·5	71
Gall-bladder or liver trouble	44·4	36·1	8·3	11·1	36

stomach upset were most common in social classes I, II, and III; very poor appetite, diarrhoea, and weight change were all most often reported by persons in social class III. Whereas complaints of very poor appetite and weight change were most often reported by the separated and divorced (13 per cent and 15 per cent respectively of the separated and divorced), diarrhoea was commonest among the single (57 per cent) and indigestion among the married (23 per cent). The unemployed reported most complaints of weight change (13 per cent of the unemployed), very poor appetite (31 per cent), and indigestion (33 per cent), in which last complaint they were closely followed by the retired (31 per cent). Diarrhoea was most often complained of by the retired.

Reporting of each of these complaints rose with the total number of complaints reported by each person. There was very little variation in rates of reporting according to household size.

WHO MADE THE DIAGNOSIS

Surprisingly few of these complaints had been medically diagnosed, as is shown in *Table 27*.

TABLE 27

Digestive complaints according to who originally made the diagnosis

| Complaints | Who diagnosed | | Total |
	Doctor	Other	(=100%)
Indigestion, heartburn, nausea, vomiting	17·4	82·6	374
Stomach upset, gastro-enteritis	30·1	69·9	236
Very poor appetite	11·0	89·0	173
Diarrhoea	14·1	85·9	71
Big loss in weight	18·9	81·1	53
Dental disorder	100·0	—	52
Blood in bowel motions	37·5	62·5	24
Obesity	40·0	60·0	10
Hernia or rupture	88·9	11·1	9
Stomach, peptic, or duodenal ulcer	85·7	14·3	7
Gall-bladder or liver trouble	66·7	33·3	3
Total	22·7	77·3	1012

Very few of the social factors collected were significantly correlated with whether or not digestive disorders were taken to the doctor. In the case of indigestion, significantly more complaints by those aged over 60 years (32 per cent of all complaints in these age-groups) and by those aged 30–39 years (25 per cent) were taken to the doctor. The chi-square test was significant at the 0·01 level. The same level of statistical significance was reached in the correlation of employment status with indigestion, where the retired most often consulted the doctor (36 per cent of the retired with this complaint) followed by housewives (24 per cent), the unemployed (23 per cent), and the employed (15 per cent). Complaints of very poor appetite were significantly (chi-square significant at the 0·05 level) more likely to be taken to the doctor as the total number of complaints rose, and weight change was significantly (at the 0·01 level) more likely to be taken if only a small number of complaints was experienced.

Multiple regression analysis showed that in the case of complaints of changes in weight, 9·8 per cent of the difference between those who had ever consulted a doctor and those who had not was explained by the total number of all complaints reported, and a further 4·9 per cent by age. When all variables were considered, the percentage of difference explained was 17 per cent. For anal complaints (excluding complaints of blood in the bowel motions) 9·2 per cent of the difference was explained by sex. When all seven of our variables were taken into account the percentage of difference explained rose to 16 per cent. Differences between the two groups in respect of complaints of diarrhoea were explained up to 4·2 per cent by household size and an additional 6 per cent by sex. All variables together explained 12 per cent of the difference.

Differences between the two groups in complaints of indigestion and of very poor appetite were much less well explained. In the case of indigestion, age explained 2 per cent of the difference, and all variables together 3 per cent. The difference for those complaining of a very poor appetite was explained to the extent of 2·4 per cent by age, and consideration of all variables raised this to 4·4 per cent.

ACTION TAKEN

Table 28 shows the action taken for these complaints (with the exception of medicine) during the fourteen days before interview.

Of the 43 complaints (4·2 per cent of all digestive complaints) that had received medical care, 27 had been taken to the doctor in his surgery. The next largest group (7 persons) had been visited by a doctor in their own homes. A further 7 had been to hospital, 3 to an outpatient clinic, and 4 had been inpatients. The local authority had looked after two patients at a London County Council clinic. Of the 14 complaints for which advice had been asked of a non-medical person, 10 had been referred to a chemist and 4 to a lay person.

During the fourteen days before interview, 49 persons had visited a general dental practitioner and 3 had been to see a dentist at a hospital.

TABLE 28

Action taken for digestive complaints over a 14-day period

Action	No.	%	As a percentage of all these complaints
Sought medical care*	43	50·0	4·2
Stayed away from work	15	17·4	1·5
Went to bed	14	16·3	1·4
Asked non-medical advice	14	16·3	1·4
Total	86	100·0	8·5

* Does not include dental care.

TABLE 29

Percentage of digestive complaints for which medicines were taken, and who prescribed them

Complaint	Percentage of complaints medicated Doctor*	Other	Total no. of complaints
Indigestion, heartburn, nausea, vomiting	12·8	43·0	374
Stomach upset, gastro-enteritis	22·5	56·4	236
Very poor appetite	5·2	7·5	173
Diarrhoea	5·6	21·1	71
Big loss in weight	3·8	1·9	53
Dental disorder	9·6	7·3	52
Blood in bowel motions	8·3	8·3	24
Obesity	70·0	10·0	10
Hernia or rupture	33·3	11·1	9
Stomach, peptic, or duodenal ulcer	71·4	—	7
Gall-bladder or liver trouble	—	—	3
Total	138 (13·6%)	365 (36·1%)	1012 (100%)

* In the case of dental disorder this includes both medical and dental prescription.

Whereas only 43 of these complaints had actually been dealt with by some medical-care agency in the fourteen days before interview, half of them – 503 or 50 per cent – were being medicated, as is shown in *Table 29*. The higher percentage of complaints of indigestion, heartburn, nausea, and vomiting (56 per cent) were being medicated, as were 80 per cent of complaints of obesity, 79 per cent of complaints of stomach upsets and gastro-enteritis, and 71 per cent of stomach, duodenal, and peptic ulcers. There was almost three times as much lay as medical medication.

The most commonly used medicines were antacids, followed by other measures – most often the use of a special diet – analgesics and salts. Of all digestive disorders 3 per cent were being medicated by respondents themselves as well as by their doctors, and 3 per cent were being treated with more than one lay-prescribed medicine at the same time. (See also Appendix II, *Table D*.)

ATTRIBUTED CAUSES

With the exception of complaints of tiredness, worry, nervousness, and headaches, digestive complaints were the group of disorders most commonly said to have been the result of a psychological problem, and 16 per cent of doctors' diagnoses and 5 per cent of lay diagnoses were reported as assigning psychological causes. Otherwise, of all lay-diagnosed complaints, 77 per cent were reported as being the result of physical causes and 18 per cent were thought to have been caused by environmental factors. The corresponding figures for doctor-diagnosed complaints were 83 per cent due to physical causes and 1 per cent to environmental causes.

SUMMARY

Females more often than males reported digestive complaints. The age-group 30–49 years was that in which most reporting occurred. Persons in social classes I, II, and III reported proportionately more of these disorders than those in other social classes. The unmarried and persons not employed had a greater tendency to report these complaints, as did persons with a higher total number of complaints.

Of all these disorders, 23 per cent had at some time been taken to a doctor. Factors correlating significantly with seeking medical care were membership of the age-groups 30–39 years or 60 + years, not being employed, and having certain numbers of complaints. In the fourteen days before interview, doctors had been consulted about 4 per cent of these complaints, and 50 per cent of them were being medicated, a quarter of these with medicines prescribed by a doctor.

REFERENCES

1. ACHESON, H. W. K. (1962) *Morbidity Statistics from General Practice.* **5** 67. HMSO, London.
2. FRY, J. (1964) General Practice Tomorrow. *Brit. med. J.* **2** 1065.

CHAPTER 9

Skin Complaints

In this survey about one-tenth of the consultations taking place in the doctor's surgery were concerned with lesions of the skin. During the year about one-fifth of the patients who came to consult him came because of skin lesions on at least one occasion.'[1] Thus begins a chapter on skin diseases in the report of a study made by the General Register Office and the (then) College of General Practitioners into the distribution of skin disease as seen in general practice.

This indication of frequency of occurrence is supported regularly each year by the statistics of absence from work due to skin disease. The connection between various occupations and skin disorders (for example, the many varieties of contact dermatitis) is too well known to be mentioned here in any detail. However it does seem important to remember that many of the working males in the population studied are dockers, transport workers, and warehousemen concerned with the loading and unloading of all sorts of materials, among them cement, timber, and several varieties of grain and meal feeding-stuffs.

For purposes of comparison with the figures given above it may also be helpful to quote estimates of incidence of chronic skin disease. 'About 2 per cent of the population are believed to have psoriasis [2] so that the average general practitioner will have about 50 such patients in his care. Psoriasis is also common in hospital practice: it accounts for 8–9 per cent of all new attendances in this department.'[3]

In this study the 502 skin complaints were the fifth most common group and constituted 5 per cent of all complaints. *Table 30* shows details of each complaint in this group. Whereas specific questions were asked about itching, burning, rash, psoriasis, and other long-standing skin trouble all other information recorded in this table was volunteered by respondents, which probably accounts for the very low numbers of complaints of corns and callosities. *Table 31* gives the reported states of activity of the 106 chronic complaints.

TABLE 30

Grouped skin complaints relating to a 14-day period

Complaint	No.	%
Boils, impetigo, eczema, dermatitis, pruritis	244	48·6
Itching, burning, rash	170	33·9
Corns and callosities	55	10·9
Other long-standing skin trouble	32	6·4
Psoriasis	1	0·2
Total	502	100·0

TABLE 31

Activity states of reported chronic skin complaints

Complaint	Cleared up by itself or with treatment	Active at present	Still active but no symptoms in last 14 days	Total (= 100%)
Psoriasis	55·6	11·1	33·3	9
Other long-standing skin disease	39·2	33·0	27·8	97

WHO REPORTED THESE COMPLAINTS

Complaints of skin disease of all kinds were commonest in the age-groups 21–29 and 30–39 years, and were reported by 32 per cent of respondents. Reporting rates declined with increasing age. Females outnumbered males in reporting skin disorder for all apparently minor conditions but were outnumbered by males in reporting chronic conditions. It was interesting to see that for females reporting of corns and callosities began in the youngest group with 32 per cent, and fell with increasing age, which probably indicates that the younger female had not yet learnt to 'live with' these complaints.

Reporting of skin complaints was commonest from social classes I and II (31 per cent), and declined very slightly (to 26 per cent) with descending social class. It was also more frequent from single (32 per cent) and married (27 per cent) persons than from the widowed separated, and divorced (23 per cent). Those unemployed reported more often (33 per cent) than persons in other employment states who all gave very similar rates (27 per cent).

WHO MADE THE DIAGNOSIS

Table 32 indicates who originally had diagnosed the condition reported. Consulting a doctor about skin disease was only significantly associated with being unemployed (chi-square significant at the 0·001 level), and 46 per cent of the unemployed had at some stage had their skin complaints medically diagnosed.

TABLE 32

Skin complaints according to who originally made the diagnosis

Complaint	Who diagnosed Doctor	Non-medical	Total (=100%)
Boils, impetigo, eczema, dermatitis, pruritis	29·1	70·9	244
Itching, burning, rash	19·4	80·6	170
Corns and callosities	—	100·0	55
Other long-standing skin trouble	68·8	31·2	32
Psoriasis	100·0	—	1
Total	27·3	72·7	502

Multiple regression analysis showed that our seven chosen variables were of least value in explaining the difference between those who went to the doctor and those who did not in the case of skin complaints. Unemployment and the total number of complaints reported together explained only 2 per cent of the difference, and when all variables were taken into account 3·2 per cent of the difference was explained.

ACTION TAKEN

Table 33 shows the four main types of measure resorted to during the fourteen-day period before interview. It shows that these conditions were unusual in that, although 25 of them were taken to medical care, for 6 complaints lay advice was asked. It was also interesting to find that as many as 11 of these complaints had merited time away from work. Two complaints had been dealt with by a chiropodist, and 3 had been taken to an outpatient department. An industrial medical officer had attended to one complaint, eighteen had been taken to a general practitioner, and in two cases the doctor had visited a respondent at home.

TABLE 33

Action taken for skin complaints over a period of 14 days

Action	No.	As a percentage of these complaints
Sought medical care	26	5·2
Stayed away from work	11	2·2
Asked non-medical advice	6	1·2
Went to bed	4	0·8
Total	47	9·4

TABLE 34

Percentage of skin complaints for which medicines were taken and who prescribed them

Complaint	Percentage of complaints medicated		Total no. of complaints
	Doctor	Other	
Boils, impetigo, eczema, dermatitis, pruritis	25·4	64·8	244
Itching, burning, rash	8·2	28·8	170
Corns and callosities	—	54·5	55
Other long-standing skin disease	37·5	50·0	32
Psoriasis	100·0	—	1
Total	89 (17·7)	253 (50·4)	502

Table 34 shows that two-thirds (68 per cent) of all skin complaints were being medicated. Lay medication exceeded medical prescription, for all individual complaints except the one case of psoriasis. The most commonly medicated complaint (excluding the case of psoriasis) was the general category of boils, impetigo, etc., where 90 per cent of complaints were being medicated. Most commonly self-medicated were also boils and impetigo (65 per cent) and the most frequently medicated

by a doctor (again excluding psoriasis) were complaints of long-standing skin disease (38 per cent). Regardless of who had made the prescription, the widest range of medicines used was for the boils, impetigo, etc. group. Sixty-four different types of skin medicine were being used, and a number of other measures also, such as cutting corns and rubbing spittle into them. One man (a welder) cauterized himself following a laceration at work.

Lader found that of a population of 207 patients, both male and female, 2·2 per cent had self-medicated skin complaints during the year preceding interview.[4] Of all skin complaints in the present study, 32 per cent received no kind of medication, and they were chiefly those less specifically described, that is, itching, burning, and rash. (See also Appendix II, *Table E*.)

ATTRIBUTED CAUSES

Doctors were most often reported as attributing skin disease that they had diagnosed as being the result of physical causes (74 per cent of doctors' diagnoses), followed by the environment (16 per cent) and by psychological causes (10 per cent). Respondents themselves cited environmental causes in 67 per cent of lay-diagnosed complaints, physical causes in 31 per cent of these cases, and psychological causes in 2 per cent. Environmental causes were largely clothing, cosmetics, and the weather; work and housework accounted for only 12 per cent of these causes.

SUMMARY

Skin complaints were proportionately more often reported by the younger age-groups, with males outnumbering females in reporting more serious skin complaints and vice versa. Reporting was slightly more common by social classes I and II, by single persons, and by the unemployed.

Unemployment was the only factor significantly associated with consulting a doctor, and altogether 27 per cent of skin complaints had at some time been diagnosed by a doctor. Of all these disorders, 5 per cent had been taken to a doctor in the two weeks before interview and 68 per cent were being treated with some kind of medication. It was reported that doctors were more inclined to attribute those complaints which they had seen to physical causes than were lay persons making their own diagnoses, who more frequently cited environmental factors as causative.

Multiple regression analysis showed unemployment and the total number of all complaints reported to be the most important factors in explaining the difference between those ever consulting medical care with these complaints and those not doing so, but they accounted for only 2 per cent of the difference. All variables taken together explained 3·2 per cent of the difference.

REFERENCES

1. GRANT, R. M. R. (1962) *Morbidity Statistics from General Practice* III, p. 73. HMSO, London.
2. INGRAM, J. T. (1953) *Brit. med. J.* **2** 591.
3. SHUSTER, S. & COMAISH, J. S. (1966) The Problem of Psoriasis. *Practitioner* **196** 621.
4. LADER, SUSAN (1965) A Survey of the Incidence of Self-Medication. *Practitioner* **194** 132.

CHAPTER 10

Conclusions

SUMMARY OF FINDINGS

The aim of this study has been to describe what medicines and measures were being taken by a randomly selected population of adults to manage their health complaints. This investigation was seen as a first step in the study of demand for medical care. There were two indications of the need for an investigation of this kind, one clinical and epidemiological, and the other administrative.

The clinical and epidemiological reasons, which are intimately connected with changes in population structure mentioned in the Introduction, may be summarized by reference to two models concerning some aspects of the shifting pattern of disease. The first, the *iceberg concept*, states – very crudely – that there is a pool of unrecognized illness that is greater in proportion than the amount of illness managed, at any one time, by medical care. The amount of 'below the surface illness' varies between diseases and with the sensitivity of diagnostic methods used in screening examinations. The second, the *onion principle*, is closely connected. It states that for the community a condition of absolute health is impossible, for as one predominating set of illnesses is brought under control (for example, tuberculosis) so another 'layer' (for example, mental illness) is revealed. The administrative reasons are concerned with complaints, from many general practitioners and others, that doctors are overwhelmed with trivial complaints at a time when there is an apparent shortage of medical manpower.

The findings showed that, of a total study population of 2,153 adults, 5 per cent of persons reported no complaints during the fourteen days before interview, 19 per cent reported complaints but had taken no action about them, and 76 per cent were taking action for current complaints. Although 32 per cent of respondents had consulted a doctor at some stage (not necessarily in the fourteen days before interview) about their complaints, a quarter (26 per cent) had not seen a doctor for between one and four years. On average, during the 14-day recall period, males had taken 1·9 medicines, and females 2·2 medicines. The five most common complaints and their management are summarized in *Table 35*.

TABLE 35

Summary of management of the five most common groups of complaints, expressed in each case as a percentage of all complaints in that group

Complaint group	Visted a doctor *	Away from work *	Bed rest *	Asked non-medical advice *	Medically prescribed medication *	Non-medically prescribed medication *	Who had ever diagnosed Medical	Non-medical
Respiratory	4·1	3·0	1·0	0·6	13·0	21·1	37·0	63·0
Tiredness, worry, etc.	3·7	1·7	0·8	0·3	11·1	19·0	19·6	80·4
Rheumatic	5·1	1·6	1·0	0·1	16·4	29·8	39·2	60·8
Digestive	4·2	1·5	1·4	1·4	13·6	36·1	22·7	77·3
Skin	5·0	2·2	1·2	0·8	17·7	50·4	27·3	72·7

* During the previous 14 days.

Our analysis showed that, although the seven variables (age, sex, marital status, social class, employment status, household size, and total number of complaints) used to classify each respondent were of descriptive value and significance – and they were originally chosen only for this purpose – they explained only a relatively small percentage of the difference between those who had consulted the doctor and those who had not. This was not surprising in view of the nature of the variables. The value of the attempt to explain this difference is to be found in its emphasis on two points: namely that the most significant explanatory variables varied as between complaints, and that social class was rarely of importance. Both of these points are emphasized by the descriptive work, and they help to throw light on some of the hypotheses outlined in Chapter 2.

That social class was rarely of importance in explaining some aspects of our findings, and that the multiple regression analysis accounted for a very small percentage of the difference between those persons with complaints who had sought medical care and those who had not, both support recent contention that sound explanations of this difference are not to be found in simple and readily available descriptive variables concerning social position, but are more likely to lie in the more complex areas of social interaction and role. At first sight this may appear to reduce considerably any hopes for easy prediction of who will be more likely to seek medical care and who less likely, but even in these areas might there be more accessible measures that could hint at proneness to consult? Our common descriptive findings that the divorced, widowed, and single, and the unemployed as well as housewives and the retired, more often take certain complaints to the doctor than are taken by the married and the employed may be an indicator that such measures exist, although, as the multiple regression analysis showed, their predictive value was in this case of low yield.

More positively, our findings lead us to agree with Gordon that 'for all socio-economic groups, the major factor in defining someone as sick appears to be prognosis'.[1] It seems to us that the nature of the complaints themselves will be of considerable significance in the individual's decision about seeking medical care, and that if this is so then differences in consultation rates should be found between groups of complaints. We found this to be the case in our population sample, and it is discussed in greater detail later in this chapter.

COMPARISON WITH TWO OTHER STUDIES

In 1969, after the fieldwork for the present investigation was completed, an interim report was published about the work of a screening clinic organized by the Medical Officer of Health in the Greater London Council Borough of Southwark, which includes all the areas where the original study population lived. In this screening study a battery of tests was administered to a population aged 16–60 years and of both sexes.[*][2] Tests were carried out in a specially converted caravan which was taken to various parts of the borough during the four months of the study. All homes in the vicinity were visited, and persons of suitable age invited, by health visitors and nursing staff, to attend for a health check.

* The survey consisted of the following tests. A social history, a medical history, a haemoglobin estimation, blood-pressure test, urine test, measurement of height and weight, vision test, cervical smear offered to women over 25 years, general physical examination, X-ray of chest.

Comparison between this study and our own is especially interesting in view of the similarity of the populations concerned. *Table 36A* shows the age and sex distribution of the two study populations, and *Table 36B* the distribution of social class. The comparative deficit of males in the screening study population is probably due to the fact

TABLE 36A

Comparison of the two study populations by age and sex

	The present study		Southwark screening study		
Age	*Males*	*Females*	*Males*	*Females*	*Age*
21–39	23·0	21·7	10·8	43·8	16–40
40–59	26·8	28·5	10·5	34·9	41–60
Total	49·8	50·2	21·3	78·7	*Total*

Guy's 100% = 1,580　　　　　　Southwark 100% = 1,000

TABLE 36B

Social class	The present study	Southwark screening study
I	0·7	1·4
II	4·9	14·4
III	50·0	51·1
IV	25·1	16·0
V	19·3	13·4
Unknown	—	3·7
Total (= 100%)	2,153	1,000

that no evening clinic sessions were held, and is therefore unlikely to indicate accurately the level of demand.

Table 37 presents a summary of findings of the two investigations, with complaints divided into three groups. In group I, which consists of diseases of the respiratory system and diseases of the bones and organs of movement, whichever of the three methods of disposal of a complaint obtained, the doctor was presented, of the patient's own volition, with the largest percentage of complaints. A second group is made up of two conditions – mental, psychoneurotic, and personality disorders, and skin disorders – of which the largest percentages were not presented to the doctor. The third group consists of disorders that were largely discovered at the screening examination.

There are, of course, a number of difficulties in the comparison of these data. First, in the classification of disorders. Although the International Standard Classification Code was used, only the first and third columns of *Table 37* are strictly comparable. This is because they are both made up of information assessed and categorized by

TABLE 37

Comparison of findings of the present study with those of the Southwark screening study

Classification of complaints	Disorders found in Southwark screening study	The present study			
		All complaints reported	Diagnosed by a doctor	Lay-diagnosed	Total for cols. 3 and 4 (=100%)
	1	**2**	**3**	**4**	
Group I					
Respiratory	4·1	27·7	37·0	63·0	2,397
Bones and organs of movement	7·0	16·6	39·2	60·8	1,433
Group II					
Mental and psychoneurotic	7·6	22·8	19·6	80·4	1,968
Skin	3·3	5·8	27·3	72·7	502
Group III					
Digestive (includes weight change)	23·2	11·7	22·7	77·3	1,012
Nervous system	23·5	8·3	40·9	59·1	719
Metabolic and endocrine, etc.	0·3	0·1	70·0	30·0	10
Circulatory	12·8	4·5	42·0	58·0	393
Breast	0·2	0·01	100·0	—	1
Gynaecological and genito-urinary	17·9	2·4	23·6	76·4	208
Total complaints (=100%)	2,171	8,643			

doctors, whereas column 4 is a lay description of complaints. Thus, for example, as discussed at greater length in Chapter 4, a lay complaint of backache might well be coded as a disorder of the bones and organs of movement, but after assessment by a doctor it might be diagnosed as a disorder of the genito-urinary system.

Second, the tests used at the screening examination may very well not have covered in every way all manifestations of disorder possible within each disease group. This is evident from the fact that, although respiratory complaints accounted for only 4·1 per cent of all disorder discovered at screening, in our study 32·6 per cent of complaints presented to the doctor were of respiratory disease.

In the present study the proportions of persons with no complaints or diseases reported was 4·9 per cent, and in the Southwark screening study it was 6·7 per cent. Altogether, 52 per cent of persons screened were found to be in need of further investigation and possibly treatment.

IMPLICATIONS OF THE FINDINGS

It is sometimes said that some of the complaints presented nowadays to general practitioners are the sort of things that, in the days before the National Health Service, would have generally been thought too trivial to take to a doctor. Nevertheless, it is evident from our data that the use of lay-prescribed medicines and measures was a very common occurrence in the study population, and in the report of the Southwark screening study a large number of persons (51·9 per cent of the study population) were classified as referred for 'further investigation and possible treatment'. Of course, some of these cases referred after screening might not have been complaining of their symptoms, but would be sent for diagnosis. In our study there is no evidence to show whether lay medication was carried out because complaints were too trivial, or whether respondents had some other reason for not having recourse to medical care, but it is clear that the ready and free availability of medical treatment does not necessarily eradicate lay diagnosis and management.

It is important to remember that the prevailing pattern of disease is changing in such a way that chronic disorders are coming very much to the fore, and that these, by their very nature, inevitably bring with them a different pattern of consultation. *Figure 3A* illustrates this. It shows diagrammatically a typical course of the now relatively less prevalent acute disease. In a very short space of time the sufferer passes from a state of feeling healthy to feeling unwell, and he recognizes that he is ill soon after the disease process begins. Rapidly it becomes clear that he really is ill. Most of the infectious diseases provide examples of this kind of acute illness.

Figure 3B, on the other hand, shows a typical course of the kind of illness that is becoming more and more common. Here the time scale is considerably increased. Deviations from a normal state of health are small, and may appear quite trivial. For example, an outcrop of boils, an unexplained bout of indigestion, or transient giddiness may

Figures 3A and 3B   An illustration of the course of acute and episodic disease in the individual

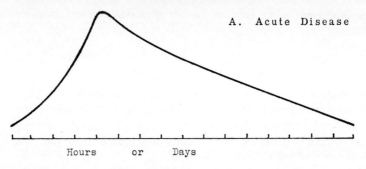

A. Acute Disease

Hours   or   Days

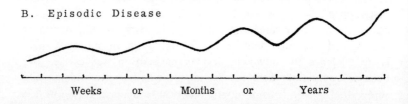

B. Episodic Disease

Weeks   or   Months   or   Years

be tolerated for years. For some pleope such incidents may be sufficiently disruptive to warrant consulting the doctor, for some it is perhaps easier to buy a tonic or an antacid remedy, and others just adapt life to handle these events; for example, they may avoid fatty foods, or go to bed earlier. Whichever course of action is chosen – doctor, chemist, or self-medication – it is common, in this type of chronic illness, for incidents of this kind to disappear as insidiously as they come. We suggest that the *episodic* pattern of many of the common diseases of today predisposes some people to lay medication, or to ignore apparently trivial complaints, so that the point of recourse to medical care is pushed much further on into the course of the manifest illness itself. This is, of course, true not only for lay persons, but also for doctors, who sometimes find that only when looking back after a diagnosis has been made does the meaning of a pattern of different symptoms presented over a period of time become explicable.

It is therefore not so surprising that we should have found such a large number of complaints. Nor is it surprising that there are so many complaints from general practitioners of 'trivia' being presented at their surgeries.

These descriptive findings all point to the necessity for an understanding of the significance of lay diagnosis and treatment, which, in view of some of the foregoing observations and of many intervening factors, such as high-pressure advertising, seem unlikely to diminish. If Morris's statement that 'Needs have to be felt as such, perceived, then expressed in demand'[3] is correct, then the period of lay diagnosis and treatment is of great importance, and this is true whether it occurs before presentation of a complaint to medical care, or during a course of medical treatment, or following it. The sufferers' interpretation of symptoms determines the threshold of complaint, the point at which it becomes demand for medical care. In any event, lay diagnoses and treatments fall into two types. First (a) those relating to symptoms that are recognized or suspected by the sufferer as needing medical care, and second (b) those relating to symptoms that are believed to indicate merely a minor complaint.

(a) *Complaints suspected of needing medical care*

In the first case it is clear that a study of those individuals who seek medical care very late in an illness (i.e. have for that set of complaints a high threshold of consultation) would be important. In the present study, fear of investigation and of treatment were cited by some respondents as reasons for not going to the doctor. In a similar way, others said that the long wait at the doctor's, and the risk of 'catching things' while waiting, made it better to treat oneself. Some respondents had not consulted their doctors again because they said nothing could be done for their complaint; for some this was a conclusion reached of their own accord and for some it was the result of a previous medical consultation. Complaints of nervousness and depression were often referred to in this way. The elderly and persons with a complaint very commonly experienced in the two boroughs (e.g. lorry drivers with backache, and dockers with lumps in the groin) were sometimes prepared to look after themselves because they felt that their complaint was inevitable at their age or in their occupation. Thus, impressionistically, it seems not only that fear of both social and physical consequences contributes to the delayed consultation but, as Morris has suggested, that the nature of the service also plays a part. Social acceptability or otherwise of a complaint (i.e. whether it is regarded as a normal condition in the circumstances or not) is important too. It may well be that 'when illness is of a kind that is common and familiar, and the course of the illness is predictable, the presentation of the illness for medical scrutiny is substantially related to an index of inclination to use medical services'.[4]

Perhaps there is also a common bias in attitudes towards some kinds of complaint. Just as in the nineteenth century poverty was thought of as 'evidence of social demoralization . . . which implies not only want of resources, but usually on the moral or physical side the want of some of the qualities that are essential to sustain life in a civilised community',[5] so it may be that present attitudes towards indications of mental stress and illness or 'being unable to cope' help to delay consultations by individuals suffering physical complaints often thought to have such origins.

Since the examples given above of reasons for not seeking medical care about complaints that respondents realized were not trivial, were the result of collecting interviewers' notes, their distribution by complaint cannot be plotted. Nevertheless, we think that there is an association in some instances between threshold of consultation and the nature of the complaint itself. For example, although no suitable data were collected, the impression is that some persons interviewed who complained of digestive disorder had consulted, or intended to consult, a doctor as late as possible in the course of their complaint. We believe that further research concentrating on this point will show trends towards late consultation by particular groups in the population for certain complaints, and that the findings will prove to be of some use in preventive medicine.

(b) *Complaints thought by the respondent to be trivial*

The second group of complaints classifiable as possibly demonstrating 'need' are those where ignorance or misunderstanding acted as a hindrance to their reaching medical care. In this situation the individual is either unaware of the seriousness of his complaint and/or is treating himself in some potentially harmful way. The present study had no means of calculating the first situation, but has demonstrated the existence of the second. To draw examples specifically from one set of complaints, namely digestive disorder, analgesics, among them very often aspirin, were commonly used in complaints of poor appetite, of indigestion, and of gastro-enteritis. Laxatives, purgatives, and ointments were used for complaints of blood in the bowel motions, respiratory medicines for diarrhoea, and counter-irritants for gastro-enteritis. Although the need for much more health education is self-evident and the necessity for more precise instructions to be enclosed with all patent medicines is indicated by such examples, at the same time all lay medication should not be condemned out of hand. It is quite possible that in some cases it is of important psychological benefit.

SUMMARY

It seems, from work on the changing pattern of disease, that the common diseases now often have an insidious onset and an episodic course, and, that this is a pattern which we have to accept with all its implications. We now have to decide how to make the best of a situation where definitive decisions about disease are very often difficult to make, both for the doctor and for the layman. Consequently a number of questions arise for the practising doctor, for the research worker both in medicine and in social science, for the medical administrator, and for the medical planner.

First, the research questions. As the common disease processes tend increasingly to be on a longer time scale, much more needs to be known about the natural history of their early stages. Work is, of course, being carried out on these problems, especially in conjunction with the development of screening techniques. At the same time, some kind of systematic National Health Survey, rather like the US National Health Survey, needs to be undertaken at regular intervals, perhaps once every five years. This is essential if we are to keep a check on the usefulness of continuing screening methods. At the present time, for example, after several years of intensive screening in many populations both routinely by general practitioners and by specially mounted studies, the numbers of previously undetected diabetics discovered in screening projects are falling. They may eventually reach a level where effort in screening for this disease would be better directed to another condition, and it is obviously important to know when this level is reached; for the same reason the decision to curtail Mass Miniature Radiographical examination is already being taken.

From the social sciences, an important contribution will be made by investigating the earliest processes of self-referral to medical care, and the acceptance of offers of screening, and particularly by eliciting reasons for refusal. This would help to give a better understanding of such problems as the apparent bias in consultation patterns for some conditions, and thus be of assistance in planning future services. Further research is indicated into self-medication; at least one large study is already being undertaken in this country[6] to investigate not only the extent of self-medication but also, for the first time, the amount of medicines present in homes, means used to dispose of medicines prescribed for a condition now cleared up, and methods of storing medicines.

Finally, a number of points may be made that are relevant to practising doctors, to medical administrators, and to planners. Essentially, our main point is that services need to change to cope with changes in disease patterns. It is clear from many studies that modern diagnostic thinking has to be very readily adaptable to changes in the prevailing disease pattern, and that such changes therefore need to be carefully monitored. Thus, if increasing numbers of conditions are known to begin insidiously and over a long period of time, then patients' reports of apparently trivial conditions are of increasing potential clinical significance. Accordingly, two things seem necessary for the future: a fast feedback of proven information about early indicators of disease, and greater use of an improved system of record-keeping (ideally backed by record linkage) so that the relevance of a constellation of 'trivia' presented over an extended period of time is more easily recognizable.

The changes in prevailing types of illness also have important implications for the employment of paramedical staff. The need for paramedical help in 'front-line care' is clear, but it is equally clear that sharing of workload in order to free the doctor to tackle 'real' illness, leaving the more apparently 'trivial' work to paramedical staff should not lead to the doctor's missing an opportunity to make an early diagnosis. Essentially this is again a question of the use and importance of medical records.

CONCLUSION

We have shown the great extent of lay diagnosis and treatment, as compared with recourse to medical care, in our study population. Although we do not know whether this pattern holds good for the population as a whole, we believe that there are indications that problems of this nature exist generally and seem likely to continue to exist, and to be of potential clinical significance. We believe that this is a problem for study both at the academic and at the Health Service level, and we hope that its investigation will contribute to what has been called the rediscovery of

'. . . the family in a medical Odyssey. . . . Diagnosis has been likened to peeling off successive layers of an onion. I insist that the opposite process is equally important: the layers have to be put back if we are to see what an onion really is. After a long preoccupation with tissues, organs, and "disease", the patient is being rediscovered and we are rediscovering, too, his family, and rediscovering the community and the environment of which they are part.'[7]

REFERENCES

1. GORDON, G. A. (1966) *Role Theory and Illness—a Sociological Perspective*. College and University Press, New Haven.
2. EPSOM, J. E. (1969) The Mobile Health Clinic – An Interim Report on a Preliminary Analysis of the first one Thousand Patients to Attend. London Borough of Southwark, Health Department.
3. MORRIS, J. N. (1967) *Uses of Epidemiology*, p. 82. Livingstone, Edinburgh.
4. MECHANIC, D., & VOLKART, E. M. (1960) Illness Behaviour and Medical Diagnoses. *J. Hlth Hum. Behav.* **1** 86.
5. BENJAMIN, B. (1964) *Public Health and Urban Growth*, p. 21. Centre for Urban Studies, London.
6. INSTITUTE FOR SOCIAL STUDIES IN MEDICAL CARE. Personal communication.
7. APLEY, J. (1964) An Ecology of Childhood. *Lancet* **2** 4.

Methodology

Since a closely detailed and accurate picture of the local population served by the hospital was required, data collection was carried out using the household interview method.

The population density of the area surrounding Guy's Hospital is high (Bermondsey 43·5 persons per acre and Southwark 76·3 persons per acre), and a large number of people live within a radius of two miles from the hospital. Thus it was possible to interview a random selection of the population without excessive travelling. The interviewers were trained over a period of three weeks in the use of a standardized questionnaire. The local general practitioners, Medical Officers of Health, hospitals, and clinics were informed of the nature of the work, and of the fact that some of their patients might be among those chosen for interview.

THE SAMPLE CHOSEN

The sampling was divided into five phases. This made it simpler to cope with coding the questionnaire data and to maintain checks on the performance of each interviewer.

Since the survey was exclusively concerned with adults (persons aged 21 years and over), a sample of 500 names was picked from the electoral register (March 1962 and later, for phases 4 and 5, March 1963) for Bermondsey and Southwark, using a table of random sampling numbers. The 500 names were stratified in such a way that the sampling fraction was the same in each of the 51 polling areas. The effect of this procedure, carried out for each of the five phases, was that a total sample of 2,500 individuals (2·7 per cent of the total electorate for 1963) was selected.

The total sample was evenly spread over the whole area and over the whole year. In addition, the addresses were allocated to the interviewers in such a way that each, in the course of each phase, covered all parts of the area.

QUESTIONNAIRE CONSTRUCTION AND ADMINISTRATION

Review of the experience of previous workers showed that the problems of adequacy of reporting fell into two groups. On one hand those concerned with the identification of factors likely to affect accuracy and fullness of reporting, and on the other those concerned with minimizing memory error.

First, it is a well-known and documented fact that certain conditions are in themselves liable to be considered not sufficiently socially acceptable to be mentioned at interview – e.g. venereal disease, illegitimate pregnancy, and even haemorrhoids.[1, 2, 3] Second, there seems sometimes to be an underlying fear or superstition among respondents that to talk of an illness increases the likelihood of its occurrence.[4, 5] Third, the dangers inherent in interviewing persons by proxy are well known.[6, 7, 8, 9] Memory errors form the other major area of difficulty. These may take the form of involuntarily or voluntarily suppressed reporting of an illness which masks the real situation. For example, it has been suggested that some absence from work on account of sickness may be a means of avoiding an intolerable work environment.[10]

Researchers have, however, concentrated less on this aspect of memory error and more on the length of time over which an optimum recall may be expected, and on various methods of stimulating recall. The US National Health Survey first suggested that recall might be stimulated by reference to action taken by the individual. In fact it took account of only those complaints 'as a result of which the person has taken one or more action'.[11] Other studies have supported this with such findings as a large differential in reporting conditions requiring only one physician's service as compared with those requiring more attention.[12] One-day hospital stays have been shown to be poorly reported[13] and episodes involving surgical treatment were found to be better reported than those requiring no surgery.[14]

The concentration of previous research effort on these areas makes it clear that health and sickness data have to be related as closely as possible to the frame of reference of the respondent if great detail is required. The method of relating health and sickness status with

Figure 4   Outline of questionnaire construction in the order of administration

General open-ended questions

↓

Check list of medicines, measures and treatments used in previous 14 days

↓

Check list of complaints experienced during previous 14 days

↓

Two questions on accidents in previous 14 days and on late effects of injuries experienced before that

↓

Check list of chronic complaints ever experienced

↓

Check list of disabilities

↓

'Socio-economic' questions

other factors was therefore used as a self-checking device within the questionnaire, and as a reliable approach to detailed information of health-care activities. The questionnaire was constructed and administered in the order shown in *Figure 4.*

Since respondents talked more readily about their health than about other personal matters, the interview began with general health questions, and went on to check lists of measures and specified conditions. Having spoken in detail about their health, respondents were understanding about the need for supplementary information. Therefore the interview finished with the list of socio-economic questions.

This choice of order proved to be of great practical value, since for many people there seems to be a frame of reference concerned with an active condition that may only be discovered either by giving them *carte blanche* to talk about their health or by using exactly their own terminology. Thus it was not surprising to find that the general questions with which the interview began together accounted for 20·8 per cent of all answers. Usually these questions established a good rapport between respondent and interviewer, and helped the respondent to feel unrestricted as to the type and the severity of symptom information required. This avoided the difficulty noted in the Baltimore Study, where a test questionnaire which restricted inquiries, both general and specific, to chronic conditions 'appeared to result in almost complete failure on the part of the respondents to report conditions characterised by only minor manifestations'.[15]

The problem of keeping the respondent acquainted with the frame of reference is particularly important when different sorts of check-lists and questions are used one after another. For this reason each list was preceded by a brief explanation of what was to follow – e.g. 'Now I would like to read a list of various things that people do about their health' – and a definition of a period of time involved – 'Did you do any of these things in the last 14 days?'

The recall period, its relationship to the time of interview and its expression as 14 days rather than 'two weeks' or 'a fortnight' were chosen because of the close accuracy of detail required, and the possibility of memory error.

'In the California Health Survey the incidence rates for acute illnesses in the periods two, three or four weeks before interview were 73 per cent, 51 per cent, and 42 per cent of the rate one week before interview. . . . In the Charlotte pre-test for the US National Health Survey which only covered the two calendar weeks before interview . . . the incidence rate in the second week before interview was 95 per cent of that for the week immediately preceding interview.'[16]

The lists of symptoms, chronic illnesses, and impairments were all concerned with specific conditions in order to keep the frame of reference within the scope of any person interviewed. Thus lists referring to parts of the body (e.g. 'Have you had any chest complaint?') such as were used in the Survey of Sickness and the Danish National Morbidity Inquiry were avoided. As has been pointed out, 'people fail to recognize their rheumatism in a question about swollen and painful joints'.[17]

The checklist of medicines and measures tended, as in the Baltimore Study, to supplement the data already gained by use of the two general questions. These questions were designed to direct the respondent's attention to the type of information required. Thus in many cases examples were given – e.g. 'Did you use any pills or tablets, aspirins, codeine, or Alkaseltzer, and so on . . .?'

The basis for many of the questions on the checklist of symptoms may be found in the Cornell Medical Index,[18] and the MRC Respiratory Questionnaire,[19] but for the purposes of the present investigation some were reworded. There were three main reasons for revision.

1 To restrict the terms of reference e.g. 'Have you ever coughed up blood?' (CMI) 'Did you cough up any blood during the last 14 days?' (Guy's).

2 To avoid the use of leading questions (i.e. questions in which the wording tends to condition the response), e.g. 'Is your appetite always poor?' (CMI) 'Had you a very poor appetite in the last 14 days?' (Guy's).

3 To give a greater possibility of more accurate information by using both lay and medical terms; for example, the four Cornell questions concerning gynaecological complaints were rephrased:

'Have you had any complaints that only women have, such as period trouble or gynaecological complaints during the last 14 days?'

Also the Cornell list of 16 chronic conditions was enlarged to ensure that the frame of reference of the respondent would be adequately covered. For example, respondents were asked if they had had rheumatism, fibrositis, lumbago, slipped disc, sciatica, rather than just one example of a description of rheumatic disease.

Revision was generally necessary in view of the present circumstances of a personal interview rather than the Cornell method, where the subject completes his own questionnaire, and in view also of the additional aid of the foregoing medicines, measures, and treatments list.

The information collected at interview was classified into one of three groups:

1 Symptoms or complaints
2 Diagnoses or causes
3 Medicines and measures

Each positive response on the checklists was first of all qualified before recording. In the case of a medicine or measure used the respondent was asked who had prescribed it. In the case of a complaint he was asked who had made the diagnosis. This information was then recorded in the appropriate section of a recording area as shown in *Figure 5*. A new recording area was available for each item

Figure 5   A recording area

(SYMPTOM OR COMPLAINT)	(DIAGNOSIS) OR CAUSE)	MEASURES TAKEN Did you do anything about it *in the last 14 days*	
How did it affect you *in the last 14 days*	What caused it?	Medicines & treatments	Other measures

of information collected at interview. Throughout the questionnaire, whatever information was given, whether in answer to a question or offered spontaneously, was used as a starting-point. When a symptom was given (e.g. a cough) the cause was asked and whether a medicine or measure had been taken. When a cause was given (e.g. bronchitis) the symptom was asked and it was also asked whether a medicine or measure had been taken. When information concerning a medicine or measure was volunteered or given as an answer, the symptom and the cause for which it had been prescribed were asked. Thus on the questionnaire form the interviewer's reaction to any information was to complete the whole recording area. In addition, a note was made of whether both the diagnosis and the prescription of medicines and measures were of lay or medical origin.

Experience with this method showed that with the different checklists an internal self-checking device had in fact been constructed. For example, those people who failed to remember taking a medicine in the previous 14 days, even after the checklist of medicines had been read, were usually either able to remember from other lists that they had had a cough (symptom) or bronchitis (diagnosis or cause). Thus the method employed of completing a whole recording area revealed that they had in fact taken a medicine.

Although total response to the questionnaire was inevitably of variable length the method of using interlinked recording areas provided a standardized presentation of interview data that had been collected in more than one way – i.e. by means of one of several checklists, specific questions, or spontaneous admission by the respondent.

THE INTERVIEW

TABLE 38

Response to the letter of introduction

Reaction to the letter of introduction	Total response	Eventually completed interview
Telephone calls making an appointment for interview, or requesting further information about survey	107	107
Letter making an appointment for interview	8	8
Letter saying that any visit would be convenient	6	4
Letter of refusal	17	16
Total response	138	135
Response rate to all (2,500) letters of introduction	5·5%	5·4%

Two or three days before the interview was planned to take place a letter of introduction and explanation was sent to the subject. In many cases it was evident at the time of interview that the letter had been improperly read or understood. However, the letter proved to be an invaluable method of establishing initial contact between the survey team and the subjects chosen for interview, as *Table 38* shows. Slightly less than half (48·5 per cent) of the interviews were completed at the first visit.

THE INTERVIEWERS

Although a total of 11 persons carried out interviewing at various times during the survey, 5 worked consistently and carried out the bulk of the field work (93·1 per cent of all interviews). The other 6 each completed less than 70 interviews. All the interviewers were aged under 26 years, and had completed, or were in course of, a university education. All were strangers to the area and lived outside it. The main interviewers each received three weeks of training and the others a little less. Training largely consisted of interviews conducted on waiting outpatients, with an observer present. Interview data were later checked against clinician's notes. This proved to be a useful method. Not only were the interviewers able to see their own bias and errors very nearly at first hand, but it also brought to light some interesting differences in the two sets of data on a case, and demonstrated the value of the questionnaire used here as a means of collecting detailed information on presenting symptoms and their management by the respondent.

THE RESPONSE RATE AND NON-RESPONDENTS

Of the 2,500 adults selected for interview, information was incomplete for 335, an overall response rate of 86·6 per cent. This figure was consistent throughout all 5 sampling phases. The high rate of response is largely due to the repeated calls and patient explanations of the interviewers, and also to the great care taken to trace people who were no longer living at the address specified in the electoral register. These persons were traced (by asking caretakers, neighbours, shopkeepers, and landlords) and interviewed if they were still living within the area.

TABLE 39

Reasons for non-response

Reason	No.	%
Moved to an address outside the area	153	45·7
Moved to an unknown address	72	21·5
Temporarily away from household on holiday	1	0·3
Temporarily away from household in hospital	3	0·9
Temporarily away from household for other reasons	3	0·9
No answer after repeated calls	6	1·8
Refusal to cooperate	45	13·4
Too ill, aged, or infirm to cooperate	4	1·2
Name unidentified in electoral register	5	1·5
Individual dead	40	11·9
House demolished	3	0·9
Total	335	100·0

In *Table 39* the category 'temporarily away from household in hospital' contains only 3 persons because, whenever possible, the individual was interviewed either in hospital or on his return. Only 4 persons were too ill or infirm to cooperate, because where possible such respondents were interviewed by proxy. Twenty-five (1·2 per cent) subjects were interviewed in this way. Ultimately 45 persons refused to be interviewed, giving an overall refusal rate of 1·8 per cent. In cases of refusal, interviewers were instructed to discover and observe as much as possible of the person and his behaviour. From the rather anomalous body of data collected in this way two common themes emerged. In almost every case persons were frightened that the interview would reveal the unsuspected presence of some serious condition. Almost all said they did not like answering questions. There was no noticeable bias in refusals towards one sex, or one (apparent) state of home conditions, but all the persons concerned were over 30 years old.

CODING AND DATA ANALYSIS

Questionnaires were coded as soon as possible after completion. Socio-economic data were precoded. All other information was coded on to a separate transfer sheet and attached to the appropriate questionnaire.

Answers given in response to a checklist question were coded using their checklist number. All other information was wherever possible coded using the International Standard Classification four-digit code. Codes were set up for non-medical diagnoses and for all medicines and treatments. The coded material was checked by people who had taken no part in either the interviewing or the coding processes, and then transferred, both from the coding sheet and from pages one and two of the questionnaire, to punched paper tape, and thence to magnetic film. Analysis was carried out with an Elliott 803 Computer, and on the University of London Computer Centre's CDC 6600 machine, for which, of course, a magnetic tape was made.

DISCUSSION

The choice of the electoral register for the sampling frame was a result of the decision to interview individuals rather than families or households. This decision was based on the fact that the object of the study was to collect information about the things people did about their health. In order to cover all the ground necessary in such an appraisal the rather complex questionnaire described in this chapter was used, and consequently interviews took a considerable time to complete. If this process had been repeated for each member of a household the risks of slap-dash interviewing and poor cooperation from respondents would increase accordingly. It was in the light of these facts and in the likelihood that the behaviour in illness of one member of a family or household would tend strongly to follow the same patterns as that of other members, that the decision to interview individuals was taken. A study of the *motivation* of behaviour, on the other hand, would require a household interview survey. Thus the widest scope of individual attitudes and behaviour available with the resources was covered.

SUMMARY

To fulfil the aim of describing all health-care activities of a population as cheaply and thoroughly as possible a questionnaire was constructed. This was based upon the idea of a self-checking device to ensure detailed collection of data from household interviews using lay interviewers with no previous experience and a minimum level of training. This method provided not only a satisfactory coverage of health-care behaviour, but also a useful format for the handling of data from records of variable length. An Elliott machine code programme has been prepared specifically to handle this questionnaire.

REFERENCES

1. US NATIONAL HEALTH SURVEY (1963) *Comparison of Hospitalization Reporting in Three Survey Procedures.* Series D-8. Public Health Service, Washington.

2. FELDMAN, J. (1960) The Household Interview Survey as a Technique for the Collection of Morbidity Data. *J. chron. Dis.* 11 535.

3. MARLOWE, D., & CROWNE, D. (1953) Social Desirability and Response to Perceived Situational Demands. *J. consult. Psychol.* 25 109.

4. MECHANIC, D., & VOLKART, M. (1961) Stress, Illness Behaviour and the Sick Role. *Amer. sociol. Rev.* 26 51.

5. MECHANIC, D. (1962) The Concept of Illness Behaviour. *J. chron. Dis.* 15 182.

6. Op. cit. US National Health Survey (1963).

7. Op. cit. FELDMAN, J. (1960).

8. US NATIONAL HEALTH SURVEY (1964) National Centre for Health Statistics. Washington.

9. Op. cit. MARLOWE, D., & CROWNE, D. (1953).

10. MECHANIC, D., & NEWTON, MARGARET (1965) Some Problems in the Analysis of Morbidity Data. *J. chron. Dis.* 18 574.

11. Op. cit. U.S. National Health Survey (1964).

12. US NATIONAL HEALTH SURVEY (1961) Health Interview Responses Compared with Medical Records. Series D-5 Public Health Service, Washington.

13. Op. cit. U.S. National Health Survey (1963).

14. Op. cit. MECHANIC, D., & NEWTON, MARGARET (1965).

15. COMMISSION ON CHRONIC ILLNESS (1957) *Chronic Illness in a Large City.* Vol. IV of *Chronic Illness in the United States.* Harvard University Press, Cambridge, Mass.

16. CARTWRIGHT, ANN (1963) Memory Errors in a Morbidity Survey. *Milbank Memorial Fund Quarterly* 41 1.

17. CARTWRIGHT, ANN (1959) Some Problems in the Collection and Analysis of Morbidity Data Obtained from Sample Surveys. *Milbank Memorial Fund Quarterly* 37 33.

18. BRODMER, K., ERDMAN, A. J., & WOLFF, H. G. (1949) Cornell University Medical College. Cornell Medical Index Health Questionnaire.

19. MEDICAL RESEARCH COUNCIL (1960) Report of the Committee on the Aetiology of Chronic Bronchitis. *Brit. med. J.* 2 1665.

Medicines used for the Five most Common Complaints

OTHER 'MEDICINES' AND MEANS

'Medicines' in this context are substances that are not properly so defined, but were being used as such, for example various herbs, alcohol, salt, and milk. Also included are various dietary foods, such as Complan, Bovril, and Bengers Food.

'Means' includes such activities as cutting corns with a razor blade, having a Turkish bath, doing various exercises, and wearing copper bracelets for protection against arthritis.

TABLE A

Respiratory complaints

Type of medicine	Lay-prescribed medicines	Medically prescribed medicines	Total complaints for which these medicines were used = (100%)	Complaints for which these medicines were prescribed as a percentage of all these complaints (2,397)
Analgesics	93·3 (140)	6·7 (10)	150	6·3
Antacids	89·2 (33)	10·8 (4)	37	1·5
Gastro-intestinal medicines	64·3 (9)	35·7 (5)	14	0·6
Counter-irritants	50·0 (4)	50·0 (4)	8	0·3
Respiratory medicines	59·2 (210)	40·8 (145)	355	14·8
Tonics and vitamin preparations	86·7 (13)	13·3 (2)	15	0·6
Skin medicines	87·5 (7)	12·5 (1)	8	0·3
Ear and eye medicines	100·0 (1)	—	1	0·04
Medicines usually medically prescribed	13·5 (20)	86·5 (128)	148	6·2
Other medicines	85·0 (68)	15·0 (12)	80	3·3
All types of medicine	61·9 (505)	38·1 (311)	816	34·0

TABLE B

Complaints of tiredness, worry, nervousness, and headache

Type of medicine	Lay-prescribed medicines	Medically prescribed medicines	Total complaints for which these medicines were used = (100%)	Complaints for which these medicines were prescribed as a percentage of all these complaints (1,968)
Analgesics	87·6 (248)	12·4 (35)	283	14·4
Antacids	90·0 (9)	10·0 (1)	10	0·5
Gastro-intestinal medicines	84·2 (16)	15·8 (3)	19	1·0
Counter-irritants	100·0 (1)	—	1	0·05
Respiratory medicines	78·6 (22)	21·4 (6)	28	1·4
Tonics and vitamin preparations	36·4 (16)	63·6 (28)	44	2·2
Skin medicines	33·3 (2)	66·7 (4)	6	0·3
Ear and eye medicines	—	100·0 (2)	2	0·1
Medicines usually medically prescribed	7·5 (11)	92·5 (135)	146	7·5
Other medicines	90·6 (48)	9·4 (5)	53	2·7
All types of medicine	63·0 (373)	37·0 (219)	592	30·1

TABLE C

Rheumatic complaints

Type of medicine	Lay-prescribed medicines	Medically prescribed medicines	Total complaints for which these medicines were used = (100%)	Complaints for which these medicines were prescribed as a percentage of all these complaints (1,433)
Analgesics	58·5 (83)	41·5 (59)	142	9·9
Antacids	66·7 (2)	33·3 (1)	3	0·2
Gastro-intestinal medicines	92·9 (26)	7·1 (2)	28	2·0
Counter-irritants	76·7 (138)	23·3 (42)	180	12·6
Respiratory medicines	83·3 (5)	16·7 (1)	6	0·4
Tonics and vitamin preparations	50·0 (3)	50·0 (3)	6	0·4
Skin medicines	77·1 (27)	22·9 (8)	35	2·4
Ear and eye medicines	—	100·0 (3)	3	0·2
Medicines usually medically prescribed	14·3 (10)	85·7 (60)	70	4·9
Other medicines	70·4 (133)	29·6 (56)	189	13·2
All types of medicine	64·5 (427)	35·5 (235)	662	46·2

TABLE D

Digestive complaints

Type of medicine	Lay-prescribed medicines	Medically prescribed medicines	Total complaints for which these medicines were used = (100%)	Complaints for which these medicines were prescribed as a percentage of all these complaints (1,012)
Analgesics	88·1 (52)	11·9 (7)	59	5·8
Antacids	90·8 (148)	9·2 (15)	163	16·1
Gastro-intestinal medicines	91·5 (75)	8·5 (7)	82	8·1
Counter-irritants	100·0 (2)	—	2	0·2
Respiratory medicines	52·9 (9)	47·1 (8)	17	1·7
Tonics and vitamin preparations	46·7 (7)	53·3 (8)	15	1·5
Skin medicines	88·8 (8)	11·1 (1)	9	0·9
Ear and eye medicines	—	—	0	—
Medicines usually medically prescribed	8·1 (5)	91·9 (57)	62	6·1
Other medicines	62·8 (59)	37·2 (35)	94	9·3
All types of medicine	72·6 (365)	27·4 (138)	503	49·7

TABLE E

Skin complaints

Type of medicine	Lay-prescribed medicines	Medically prescribed medicines	Total complaints for which these medicines were used = (100%)	Complaints for which these medicines were prescribed as a percentage of all these complaints (502)
Analgesics	100·0 (12)	—	12	2·4
Antacids	100·0 (2)	—	2	0·4
Gastro-intestinal medicines	50·0 (2)	50·0 (2)	4	0·8
Counter-irritants	85·7 (6)	14·3 (1)	7	1·4
Respiratory medicines	—	—	0	—
Tonics and vitamin preparations	100·0 (1)	—	1	0·2
Skin medicines	76·4 (162)	23·6 (50)	212	42·2
Ear and eye medicines	66·7 (2)	33·3 (1)	3	0·6
Medicines usually medically prescribed	33·3 (14)	66·7 (28)	42	8·4
Other medicines	88·1 (52)	11·9 (7)	59	11·7
All types of medicine	74·0 (253)	26·0 (89)	342	68·1

Author Index

Acheson, H. W. K., 67, 73
Acheson, R. M., xi, xii, 25, 31
Anderson, J. A. D., 38, 43
Apley, J., 91

Balint, M., 12, 16
Barker, D. J. P., xi, xii, 25, 31
Barsky, P. N., 15, 17
Benjamin, B., 88, 91
Berg, K., 13, 17
Beveridge, W. H., 2, 4, 8
Blaney, R., xi, xii, 23, 31
Brockway, F., 22, 30
Brodmer, K., 96, 102
Brooke, E. H., 11, 15
Brotherston, J. H. F., 12, 15, 41, 43
Butterfield, W. J. H., xi, xii, 3, 8, 10, 15, 23, 25, 31

Cargill, D., 12, 15
Cartwright, A., 5, 8, 12, 15, 16, 38, 41, 43, 96, 102
Chamberlain, J. O. P., xi, xii
Clark, A. J., 12, 15
Clausen, J. A., 13, 16
Cobb, S., 14, 17
Comaish, J. S., 74, 79
Copeman, W. S. C., 60, 66
Cravioto, J., 15, 17
Crocker, L. H., 32, 43
Crowne, D., 13, 16, 93, 102

Dubos, R., 13, 16

Epsom, J. E., 11, 83, 84, 85, 91
Epstein, F. N., 6, 8

Erdman, A. J., 96, 102

Feldman, J., 93, 102
Francis, T., 6, 8
Froggatt, P., 12, 15
Fry, J., 44, 45, 51, 53, 59, 60, 66, 67, 73

Greenberg, B. G., 12, 15
Gomberg, W., 13, 17
Gordon, G. A., 14, 17, 82, 91
Grant, R. M. R., 74, 79
Gray, R. M., 13, 16

Heasman, M., 15, 17
Hinkle, L. E., 11, 15
Hollander, J. L., 60, 66
Hope, K., 12, 15
Horder, E., 12, 15
Horder, J., 12, 15

Ingram, J. T., 74, 79

Jaco, E. G., 14, 17
Jeffreys, M., 12, 15, 41, 43
Jones, H. G., 52, 59

Kadushin, C., 12, 16
Kalimo, E., 14, 17
Kesler, J. P., 13, 16
Kessel, N., 12, 15
Koos, E., 13, 16
Kosa, J., 12, 16

Lader, S., 12, 15, 78, 79
Lambo, T. A., 13, 16

107

Subject Index

medicines—*cont.*
patent, 12, 48, 89
purgatives, 89
respiratory, 57, 89, 103–5
salts, 40, 42, 49, 57, 72
sedatives, 40, 49
skin, 39–40, 49, 78, 103–5
storage in homes, 90
tonics, 40–2, 48–9, 86, 103–5
upper respiratory, 40, 49, 57
urinary, 40, 42, 49
vitamin preparations, 40–2, 48–9, 86, 103–5
mental illness, *see under* disease
metabolic disease, *see under* disease
migraine, 35
migration from the study area, 19–20
morbidity, 3–4, 9, 11–12
mortality, 19, 23
mothercraft, 28

National Health Service, 1, 2, 5, 91
expenditure on mental illness, 52
expenditure on respiratory illness, 44
expenditure on rheumatic illness, 60
expenditure on digestive illness, 67
National Health Survey, 89–90
nausea, 67–73
need for medical care, 3, 15, 87, 89
nervousness, 52–9, 88
nervous system disease, *see under* disease
neuroses, *see under* disease, menta
nurses, local authority, 83
nutritional disease, *see under* disease

obesity, 3, 10, 67–73
occupation centre, 28
old persons' homes, 28
ointments, *see under* medicines
onion principle, 3, 80, 91
operation, surgical, 13, 35, 46, 62, 68

optician, *see under* consultation
orthopaedic disorders, *see under* disease, bones and organs of movement
osteopath, 38

pain,
abdominal, 67–73
back, 11, 36, 84, 88
low back, 61–6
chest, 44–51
joint, 61–6
limb, 61–6
paramedical staff, 5, 91
Peckham Health Centre, 32
personality disorder, *see under* disease, mental
pharmacy, 3
planning, medical, 89–90
pneumonia, lobar, 3
population structure, 2, 3, 5, 80
in study area, 19–27
sample for study, 29–30, 33, 83–4, 92–3
pollution, atmospheric, 23, 44, 50
poverty, 13, 88
prediction, of demand for medical care, 2, 13–14, 82
pregnancy, 33, 36
prescribing, *see under* medication
preventive medicine, 4, 88
private practitioner, 1
prognosis, 14, 82
prolapse of the intervertebral disc, 60–6
prophylaxis, 14, 41–2
pruritis, 74–9
psoriasis, 74–9
psychiatric disorder, *see under* disease, mental
psychological causes of complaints, 42, 50, 58, 65, 72, 78
psychoneurotic disorder, *see under* disease, mental
psychosocial complaints, 14
psychosomatic complaints, 14, 52
public health measures, 9